SCHOOL HEALTH HANDBOOK

A Ready Reference for School Nurses and Educators

To my wife, Rose, whose constant encouragement, intelligent editing, and gentle nagging helped make this book a reality.

SCHOOL HEALTH HANDBOOK

A Ready Reference for School Nurses and Educators

Jerry Newton, M.D.

Director, Health Services
San Antonio Independent School District
San Antonio, Texas

Clinical Professor Pediatrics
University of Texas Health Science Center
of San Antonio

Foreword by Georgia P. Macdonough, R.N., S.N.P.

Illustrations by John Martini, MSMI

Prentice-Hall, Inc.
Englewood Cliffs, New Jersey

Prentice-Hall International, Inc., *London*
Prentice-Hall of Australia, Pty. Ltd., *Sydney*
Prentice-Hall of Canada, Inc., *Toronto*
Prentice-Hall of India Private Ltd., *New Delhi*
Prentice-Hall of Japan, Inc., *Tokyo*
Prentice-Hall of Southeast Asia Pte. Ltd., *Singapore*
Whitehall Books, Ltd., Wellington, *New Zealand*
Editora Prentice-Hall do Brasil Ltda., *Rio de Janeiro*

Library of Congress Cataloging in Publication Data

Newton, Jerry
School health handbook.

Bibliography: p.
Includes index.
1. Pediatrics—handbooks, manuals, etc.
2. School children—Diseases—Handbooks, manuals, etc.
3. Child health services—Handbooks, manuals, etc.
I. Title. [DNLM: 1. Pediatrics—handbooks. 2. School Health Services—handbooks. WS 39 N564s]
RJ48.N48 1984 618.92'0008837 84-8382

ISBN 0-13-793639-7

Printed in the United States of America

FOREWORD

Current societal and economic changes have influenced more and more parents to substantially rely on the school and its employees to monitor their children. The schools are expected not only to communicate about students' educational and social progress, but also to identify and meet their health needs.

One of the challenges to an author is to meet the needs of the readers. Jerry Newton, a physician experienced in both pediatrics and public health, has met this challenge by developing a guide that will be helpful to school nurses as well as other professional school employees.

Several characteristics mark this book as a valuable resource. First, some attention is given to administrative responsibilities in the area of school health services. This can be most helpful to persons in charge as the expertise within most school systems is in educational management and not health services. Second, the most common health conditions prevalent in the school-aged population are simply delineated with helpful hints for handling a variety of situations. Third, the line drawings accompanying this text will make the message very clear to the reader. I am sure many school children will ultimately benefit because their caretaker has access to such up-to-date, safe, and simple guidance.

Georgia P. Macdonough, R.N., S.N.P.
President, American School Health Association

ABOUT THE AUTHOR

Jerry Newton, a pediatrician with a wide variety of experiences, conducted a busy private practice in San Antonio, Texas for 23 years. This was followed by 3 years of bouncing around in a jeep as a Peace Corps physician in Paraguay, where he not only was the personal physician to 75 Peace Corps volunteers, but also the medical supervisor for the Peace Corps, Public Health Program in Paraguay.

On returning to the United States, he became the full-time medical director of the San Antonio Independent School District and has served in that position for the past 11 years. Many school districts have medical consultants but in only a few is the physician an active member of the Superintendent's staff. Moving through the corridors of 90 schools, and constant contact with school nurses, principals, and teachers, have given him an unusual insight into the special medical problems of school children and the need for better health education.

He has consistently applied his efforts to improve the quality of health care provided to students. To increase the effectiveness and expand the services provided by school nurses, he developed an active school nurse practitioner program, which has resulted in many newer and innovative school health programs, and clinics dealing with learning disabilities and behavior problems.

He is clinical professor of pediatrics at the University of Texas Medical School in San Antonio, and has been active in school health committees of his local and state medical associations as well as the American School Health Association and the American Academy of Pediatrics.

ABOUT THIS HANDBOOK

The purpose of the *School Health Handbook* is to provide a standard, well-referenced sourcebook for use by educational personnel as well as school nurses. It is written by a pediatrician with 23 years of experience in private practice and over 11 years of experience as a full-time school physician.

The need for this sourcebook has become increasingly apparent over the past decade and reflects the anxiety felt by school personnel when they are called upon to make medical decisions that will be in the best interest of their students and, at the same time, not be cause for later litigation. Budget retrenchment has forced many schools to replace nurses with lesser-trained personnel. In some cases, principals, counselors, and school secretaries find themselves without so much as a health aide, leaving medical decisions squarely on their shoulders, even though they have no medical or first-aid training. The *School Health Handbook* attempts to give them the information and guidelines required to make such decisions.

In short, this handbook is designed to serve as a "Medical Answer Book" with emphasis on what *action,* if any, school nurses or other health personnel should take when faced with specific health problems. While school nurses would understand medical terminology, school districts that do not employ nurses use nonmedical staff for the health services they may provide. So that this book will be useful to all, it is written in nontechnical language, with medical jargon either eliminated altogether or explained. The format is uniform wherever possible and provides quick answers that are easy to find.

For the user's convenience, the *Handbook* is organized into 17 sections. Section 1 deals briefly with the administrative side of school health services today. Each of the remaining 16 sections covers one major type of school health problem and begins with a short overview of section contents. Each section then covers a number of different diseases or conditions, including a description of the nature of the disorder, specific symptoms, diagnostic techniques, and guidelines for management by the school nurse or other school personnel. Some sections also include a discussion of the school relevance of the particular problem. Illustrations to supplement the information are presented.

A special "Appendix of Forms" is provided at the end of the book. The forms included are either direct examples or composites of forms actually in use in various schools. These sample forms may be copied just as they are or adapted to fit the needs of a particular school or district.

By following standardized medical procedure, as prescribed in a reliable sourcebook, school personnel should be able to justify their actions to parents, who are often not available during school hours. These actions sometimes must be defended at a meeting of the board of trustees, occasionally with the parents' attorney present. This handbook could well be used to support administrative decisions and guidelines as well as official policy of the board in matters relating to school health practices.

Special sections are included for dealing with children with severe physical disability, such as cerebral palsy and spina bifida. These will help school officials make realistic decisions about class placement and medical management as they comply with the mainstreaming requirements of P.L. 94-142, Education for All Handicapped Children.

The *School Health Handbook* should also help to increase the understanding and dialogue between doctors and teachers. Each professional has different training, a different viewpoint toward children, and different opinions concerning management of diseases and disabilities that require help from both educators and physicians. Both care deeply about the welfare of the children for whom they often share the responsibility for educational and medical management. This increased understanding should lead to better cooperation on behalf of the child whose welfare they both seek.

Jerry Newton, M.D.

AUTHOR'S NOTE

A complete school health program consists of two broad areas: Health Services and Health Education. Health Education is part of the teaching curriculum, is taught by certified teachers trained in colleges of education, and includes a wide range of health related topics. Health Services are a support service, apart from the primary educational mission of the school but necessary to the proper functioning of the complete system. Health services are provided by physicians and nurses who receive their training in medical and nursing schools.

It cannot be emphasized too strongly that these two aspects of a "complete health program" are interdependent and necessary for either part to function properly and effectively. The school child with sores in his nose and on his fingers will simply not recover very well if he does not have, through health education, some basic understanding of germs and their transmission when he picks his nose. A classroom teacher, despite her best efforts, cannot optimally instruct a child with poor vision or hearing, and it is the role of school Health Services to discover and correct these problems.

Though this book is dedicated to the provision of health services, it cannot overstate the importance of health education beginning in kindergarten as a part of the regular curriculum. There are many imaginative and interesting health education texts available that can be easily used by the regular classroom teacher.

Various forms of health services have been provided to school children for many generations in the United States, and most state education agencies require local school districts to carry on differing levels of health services activities. For example, vision screening and mandatory immunization requirements now exist in almost all states. Many states have much more comprehensive requirements; e.g., complete physical examination, neurological evaluation for special children, and followup of chronic health problems. A few school districts even provide clinics in the school itself, staffed by specially trained nurses and/or physicians. These clinics provide primary medical care to the children in that school (and sometimes neighboring schools). Children with tonsillitis, middle ear infections, skin infections, and other minor illnesses are actually diagnosed, treated, and given followup care at the same clinic. Only the more serious illnesses need be referred to a more conventional health care source.

The school primary care medical facility as described above has developed basically out of two phenomena which have been occurring in our larger and older cities: More parents are both going to work and more doctors are moving out of low-income areas. When almost all children had a nonworking parent at home, parents could be relied on to take care of the child's medical needs. Those days are over. Anybody who has taken a child to a city hospital or clinic knows that when a parent must come to school, get the child, and go to a clinic, the parent loses a full day of work. Thus, more families have come to rely on the school as a partial answer to their children's health care needs. Many school nurses already treat children with lice and scabies, though it is still the doctor who signs (or approves) the prescription for legal reasons.

It is obvious that a relatively small affluent suburban school district will require a vastly different level of school health services than an older and larger inner-city school district. Each district must develop a type of Health Services program that serves the particular needs of the children and parents in its attendance zone. The levels of health services provided should take into account community factors, such as neighborhood medical clinics, as well as school factors. Finally, if school districts must provide increased levels of health services, there should certainly be adequate funding so that educational dollars will not be diverted to health services.

CONTENTS

LIST OF ILLUSTRATIONS

SECTION 1

ADMINISTRATIVE ASPECTS OF SCHOOL HEALTH

This section briefly examines the functions of school nurses and school physicians in administering school health services and identifies some of the problems that arise with medical excuses. Standing orders and protocol are discussed, and two examples are shown. The Appendix of Forms, pages 273–291, presents a variety of administrative forms and letters that can be adapted by school nurses for use in their own school districts.

SCHOOL NURSES

Historical Background

For many years school health services have been provided by municipal health departments through the employment of city or county public health nurses. In some communities, as the demand for other public health nursing services has grown, school health services provided by municipalities have declined. In the past 20 to 30 years, many school districts have created their own departments of health services, with school nurses, supervisors, and consulting or full-time medical doctors. The school nursing profession has developed high standards and programs providing a variety of services which have become fairly well standardized throughout the states.

Relationship to School Personnel

It is important for school administrators to recognize that the school nurse's expertise is not, nor should it be, in education. Traditional school in-service programming rarely applies to the school nurse. School nurses must be given opportunities for professional renewal if they are to be of value to the school system. There are national and state organizations of school nurses, and each school nurse should be encouraged to join and to attend meetings.

Health services in most public schools are administratively separated from health education. Health service is considered a support service staffed largely by school nurses, whereas health education is part of the general education curriculum. This type of administrative arrangement tends to separate the school nurse from the formal educational process. To effectively utilize their expertise, forward-looking health educators often use school nurses as resource people when teaching about drug use and abuse, wonder drugs such as penicillin, menstruation, hygiene, nutrition, and other appropriate subjects.

The future holds great promise for an expansion of the school nurse's role. Most handicapped school children require a combination of health and education specialists. In the United States, the entire field of education, which in the past has limited itself primarily to teaching, is gradually providing ever-increasing care of handicapped children. In order to provide such health care, there will be an increasing demand for the services of school nurses.

School Nurse Functions

In addition to giving first aid in the school clinic, school nurses also perform many screening tests such as vision, hearing, height, weight, pulse, and blood pressure, on appropriate groups of children. Other functions include visits to homes and neighborhood clinics in order to follow the course of children with chronic illness. Immunizations are very important in childhood. In some school districts nurses actually give immunizations, while in others they ensure that all children have had the immunizations required by law and refer parents to where they may be obtained—at public health clinics, private doctors, and neighborhood health centers. Emerging specialized functions performed by nurses with varying degrees of advanced training are:

1. Evaluation of the medical aspects of children with learning and behavior problems. Since school nurses have both medical and educational expertise, they are able to evaluate the medical history, the socioeconomic status, the physical condition, and the relationship of all these factors to the child's learning style and behavioral pattern.
2. Special physical screening programs, such as complete physical examinations on school entry and scoliosis (spinal curvature) screening in early adolescence.
3. Special vision screening procedures in addition to the

standard visual acuity testing, such as tests for eye muscle imbalance and latent hyperopia.

4. Liaison activities between educational and medical personnel, especially in regard to special education placement, and development of the individual educational plan.

5. Medical evaluation procedures that help assess developmental levels of young children, since standard educational pencil-and-paper psychometric testing is inaccurate and difficult in very young children (ages two through four years).

Communication with the Physician

When a child has a clear-cut medical illness for which he or she is receiving adequate medical attention through the family doctor, school personnel are usually informed of the progress and nature of the disease, and there is no need for additional direct communication. However, a student may have a medical condition for which the school nurse may feel the need to talk to the doctor directly. There are two categories of such conditions:

1. Some chronic low-grade illnesses permit children to continue school attendance, but various symptoms (poor appetite, failure to play) may cause the teacher to suspect they are not doing as well as they should.
2. Some learning and behavior problems are sufficiently serious to require some form of medical intervention. In cases of this nature, school nurses often need to talk to the doctor to give input that will supplement that of the parents. In addition, the nurse is often seeking advice that will help in the child's management and education.

Because of laws governing medical confidentiality, a doctor will require written parental consent. Therefore, the nurse must talk to the parent first and obtain permission to contact the doctor. Most parents are glad to cooperate. After obtaining the necessary permission form, the nurse should mail it to the doctor. The nurse should then call the doctor's secretary, make sure the release form has arrived, and explain the nature of the call. If the above procedure is followed, the school nurse will usually receive cooperation from the doctor.

As all experienced school nurses know, things do not always go smoothly. The most serious obstacle may be an uncooperative or uncaring parent. On occasion the parent may be poorly or improperly informed.

Another problem can be an uncooperative doctor. Some doctors have very little or no familiarity with the administrative and professional operation of a school. Some medical schools and postgraduate medical training programs are beginning to incorporate some public school health experience into their programs in the hope that physicians will become better acquainted with school personnel and practices and will be more understanding of school problems.

SCHOOL PHYSICIANS

Information the Doctor Needs from School

It is usually in regard to children who have been referred for learning or behavior disorders that doctors do not understand the school's problems. Some doctors are baffled when asked to see such a child. They cannot understand why school authorities would refer a "well" child to them, and they often diagnose the child as free of disease. The child will return to school with a note saying he or she is "normal." Doctors who are knowledgeable about diagnostic procedures and management methods can be most helpful. Copies of psychometric test results, achievement tests, teacher evaluation of academic progress, and an objective narrative report of the child's behavior are essential. Also, a written two- or three-day chronological account of the child's actions over a period of an hour or two each day is necessary. This account must be strictly objective and report only the child's actions, not the observer's opinions or inferences. It should describe actions in two or three locations, such as in class, in the cafeteria, in line, or on the playground. The doctor will also need to know, in a most specific way, what the school expects from the medical evaluation—what specific deficits or defects the school hopes the doctor may be able to help ameliorate.

Sometimes the problem is simple, clear-cut, and easy to remedy. For example, a six-year-old with pure and classical attentional deficit disorder, obvious hyperactivity, and no emotional problems usually responds well to medication and presents little problem in communication between school and doctor. However, a ten-year-old who won't do his or her homework, has almost illegible handwriting, talks back to the teacher, and is one or two grade levels below his or her class in reading presents a much more difficult problem and requires a great deal of bilateral cooperation. Careful, selective neurological evaluation may reveal poor motor control, poor sequencing ability, or poor spatial arrangement ability. There may be undiscovered emotional problems that are manifested as school failure.

Choosing a Doctor

Pediatricians are most likely to be knowledgeable about and interested in school problems. Pediatric neurologists and child psychiatrists also deal in this category of disorder, but usually they see cases on referral from pediatricians or family practitioners.

If you choose a doctor by letting your fingers walk through the yellow pages, you may improve your odds slightly by considering that recently trained doctors are more apt to be knowledgeable about learning disorders and school-related problems. A pediatrician who has a special interest or extra training in behavioral or developmental pediatrics will be most helpful. Passing specialty board exams (American Board of Pediatrics, American Academy of Family Practice, etc.) and having a medical school appointment increase the chances that the doctor will be knowledgeable. You can call the office of the County Medical Society to ascertain these factors.

Beyond this, you must judge the doctor's personal qualities: returning phone calls, being available when needed, showing a genuine interest in the child, and making real efforts to help by providing sufficient time when necessary to discuss complicated problems.

MEDICAL EXCUSES

Types

The medical excuses from a doctor's office that children or their parents bring to school vary from a hastily scrawled note on a prescription slip to a formal letter. They can be categorized as follows:

1. *Excuses for acute or chronic illnesses for limited periods of time.* These periods may be long or short but in either case usually cause no school administrative problems. The school nurse knows (or can find out) that the child is legitimately ill and can suggest steps to be taken to ensure the child's continuing education.

2. *Excuses from gym class.* Some of the more common reasons doctors furnish are:

   a. Excuses for the whole school year for unspecified reasons
   b. Excuses for obesity
   c. Excuses for diseases with an emotional component, such as asthma
   d. Excuses for children who are said to catch cold easily in cold or cool weather

As a rule, doctors do not realize that physical education is a required high school course in most states. In addition, while they acknowledge the benefit of regular exercise, they do not think that missing gym classes will have a deleterious effect on a child's health. Occasionally there are emotional or psychological factors that doctor and patient feel are better kept private.

There are irregularities and injustice on both sides of this dilemma. Physicians in private practice have seen many children who had a perfectly legitimate reason for being excused from gym classes, who in one way or another received prejudicial treatment for bringing medical excuses. On the other hand, school nurses have seen many children bring hastily scrawled notes from doctors asking for a whole year's excuse for reasons that were clearly not valid.

3. *Excuses to permit change of school.* Most school districts require a student to attend the school within the geographic boundaries of the attendance zone. Usually, a medical or psychological reason contained in a note from a doctor will be considered sufficient grounds for a transfer to another school. Nevertheless, many of these transfer requests are questionable. Sometimes a child wants to go to another school to be with a friend. Sometimes the other school is near a relative where the child can go after school until the parents get home from work. The child may not want to be bused out of his or her neighborhood or into a strange one. Again, in these cases most doctors don't realize the constraints and pressures school authorities work under. Often a principal has denied a transfer request to one student and then has to justify granting one to another, especially if everyone in the neighborhood knows that the second student is not sick in any way but has a compliant physician who simply writes excuses to satisfy a demanding parent. Some excuses of this nature are justified, and some are not. It is necessary to investigate each case individually; the school nurse can help the principal in this investigation.

Action by the School Nurse

There are no easy general answers that apply to every case, but there are certain helpful guidelines:

1. Any note that excuses a child from physical education for the whole year on vague grounds should be closely questioned.
2. Ease of catching cold, mild asthma, and controlled epilepsy are not legitimate reasons for avoiding all gym classes. They *are* reasons for adapting the exercises so they are safe and not too strenuous.
3. Emotional factors are much more important; physical deformity and obesity must be considered in this category. If a

student has an honest, legitimate emotional reason for not disrobing or wearing gym clothes, and the doctor is sincerely trying to help the student, the nurse and the gym teacher should try their best to cooperate by communicating with the doctor, explaining both sides of the situation, and arriving at a satisfactory solution.

4. It is not necessary for a child to "suit up" to participate in gym class. Failure to change clothes should not lower a child's grade if the reasons are legitimate. A student can participate in an adaptive physical education program in his or her school clothes. Many middle school and high school principals condone this practice.

STANDING ORDERS AND NURSING/MEDICAL PROTOCOLS

Since almost all states have laws that prohibit nurses from making a medical diagnosis and prescribing treatment, there are differing feelings among school nurses concerning the legality of diagnosing and/or identifying obvious medical conditions or illnesses. For example, school nurses do not hesitate to identify (or diagnose) head lice; some feel competent to identify impetigo, scabies, or chicken pox, but most will not diagnose diseases such as hepatitis or scarlet fever.

In the early 1970s, for differing reasons, school nurses began to expand their scope of activities. Since then, the identification in school of conditions such as scabies, lice, impetigo, strep throat, and other minor illnesses is increasingly being done by the school nurse.

In the late 1970s, the Robert Wood Johnson Foundation funded a $5 to $6 million five-year school health project to explore the feasibility of expanding school health services. In these special school clinics, a school nurse–practitioner, under a physician's supervision, diagnoses and treats certain minor illnesses commonly seen in schools. The nurse follows protocols or a set of standing orders dated and signed by the physician supervisor. Medical and nursing practice laws permit these special arrangements in some states.

Some other school districts with part-time, full-time, or consulting physicians have developed their own sets of standing orders, not only to help the school nurse to provide more efficient health services, but also to give the nurse better legal protection. In this process each school district, with input from nurses, doctors, and school administrators, develops its own unique protocols and set of standing orders.

Listed below are conditions frequently described in school health services protocols and standing orders:

1. Abrasions
2. Acne
3. Anaphylaxis
4. Asthma
5. Blunt injury, abdomen
6. Blunt injury, chest
7. Boils
8. Burns
9. Cellulitis and lymphangitis
10. Common colds vs. allergic rhinitis
11. Conjunctivitis
12. Contact dermatitis
13. Dog bite and human bite
14. Eczema
15. Enuresis, encopresis
16. Foreign bodies
17. Head trauma
18. Herpes simplex
19. Hives, urticaria, laryngeal edema
20. Impetigo
21. Lacerations
22. Nosebleed
23. Ringworm, tinea
24. Scabies
25. Seizures, epilepsy
26. Sprain, ankle or knee
27. Sty

SAMPLE—LENGTHY AND DETAILED PROTOCOLS FOR IMPETIGO

(This type of description is often used when nurses work in relatively isolated areas and more independent decisions must be made.)

Definition

Superficial infection of the skin manifested by vesicular or pustular lesions that rapidly become crusted.

Etiology

Caused by certain strains of streptococci, staphylococcus, or by a combination of both.

Epidemiology

Can occur at any age; both sexes and all races equally vulnerable. It is often associated with poor hygiene and is contagious. Infection is spread by contact with material from skin lesions.

Clinical Manifestations

Onset usually sudden; may be prolonged with new lesions developing over several months if child is not treated.

Lesions tend to occur at site of previous injury (scratch) and at mucocutaneous junctions (corner of lip, nasal folds); common on fingers.

Red macule-vesicle-pustule-crust lesions vary in size. Multiple sites can appear readily and diffusely. Lesions are superficial because bacteria invade upper skin layers.

May have pruritus, regional adenopathy, low-grade fever.

Diagnosis

Culture of material from pustule on blood agar, rarely necessary. Lesions as described above.

Treatment

1. Antibiotic therapy for 10 days (only necessary for severe cases)
   a. Pen-Vee-K 50–100 mg/kg/day
   b. Erythromycin 20–40 mg/kg/day q.i.d. × 10 days if allergic to penicillin and no history of erythromycin sensitivity.
2. Wet compresses to crusts with careful removal t.i.d. by parent
3. Bacitracin ointment
4. Urinalysis 2–4 weeks after prescription ends or as need arises
5. Heart exam 2–4 weeks after prescription
6. Throat culture of patient and family if impetigo recurs

Prognosis

Excellent

Complications

1. Ecthyma—more serious form of impetigo with deeper invasion of streptococcus into dermis—results from neglect and poor general physical resistance.
2. Cellulitis.
3. Acute glomerular nephritis. Efficacy of penicillin therapy in preventing acute glomerular nephritis is questionable but strongly advocated at present.

Education

1. Explain carefully to parents dosage of antibiotic and importance of compliance (A.G.N.).
2. Stress importance of child's fingernails being kept short and clean.
3. Discourage scratching.
4. All involved in child's care should wash hands carefully.
5. Child's towel and wash cloth must be isolated.
6. Classmates, relatives, siblings should be observed carefully for suspicious lesions.
7. Report any change in condition (antibiotic intolerance, lesions, urinary complaints, etc.).
8. Child may attend school if under treatment for 24 hours.

Sources

1. Kemp, Silver and O'Brien, 1978, *Practical Points in Pediatrics*
2. *Olson's Whole Pediatric Catalog*

Read and approved by:

Date:

Adapted from "Protocols for Nurse Practitioner," Robert Wood Johnson School Health Project, Newburgh, New York

SAMPLE—MORE CONCISE PROTOCOLS FOR IMPETIGO

Physical findings

1. Primary lesion is a vesicle that rapidly becomes pustular.
2. Honey-colored, loosely adherent crusts.
3. Occasionally liquid or crusted pustules.
4. Most frequently found on fingers and face but may be anywhere on body.
5. Itching.
6. Contagious on direct or secondary contact.
7. Deeper lesions with thick adherent crusts called ecthyma.

Treatment

1. Bacteria live under the crusts.
2. Gently wash with soap or septisol, and remove as much of crust as possible.
3. Apply direct pressure until bleeding stops after removal of crust.
4. Apply bacitracin ointment.
5. Cover with dressing or adhesive bandage.
6. Keep fingernails short.
7. Refer moderate to severe cases to physician.
8. May attend school if under treatment.

Follow-up

1. See in clinic daily until healing process well under way.
2. Watch for cellulitis.
3. Watch for furunculosis.
4. Watch for systemic illness with fever.

Read and approved by:

Date:

SECTION 2

DISEASES OF THE SKIN

Common skin diseases covered in this section include: head lice, scabies, ringworm, impetigo, paronychia, furuncle, acne, and herpes. Included for each disease are a description of the condition and steps for its diagnosis and effective treatment.

HEAD LICE

Nature of the Condition

Because of a vast resurgence in the past ten years, head lice are probably the largest and most exasperating problem in schools today.

The head louse (*pediculosis capitis*) is about 1/16 inch long and gray. It crawls fairly fast. It cannot jump like a flea.

The adult female louse lays eggs at the base of the hair shaft right next to the scalp. The egg is then covered with a tiny bit of gelatinous material that hardens into a semi-opaque, tiny, pearly, whitish mass that is stuck tight to the hair shaft. This mass is called a nit. In about seven to ten days, the egg matures and hatches into a louse that lives by sucking blood from the scalp. Without a human host, it can live one to three days without a blood meal. Each adult lives about one to three weeks, and a female can lay eggs several times before it dies of old age.

The biggest problem with lice is *reinfestation.* The nits resist treatment and hatch live lice. Though some drug manufacturers say their products will kill nits as well as adult lice, many doctors disagree. Reinfestation from siblings and peers is a constant occurrence and is especially difficult to control when several children sleep in the same bed.

Symptoms

In severe cases one usually sees a child with long, dirty hair which is matted and unkempt. Scratching is almost always prominent. Closer inspection reveals nits and live, crawling lice.

In mild cases, the hair may appear to be clean and combed if one merely views the child from a distance. Suspicion may be aroused only because of scratching, and a close inspection may be required to see that nits or lice are present.

If lice infestation is neglected, a child's head can look pretty bad. The excessive scratching causes a secondary infection from germs normally present on the scalp (staphylococcus, etc.). These infected areas of matted hair will require frequent washing and applications of antibiotic ointment. Occasionally some of the hair must be cut away. Lymph nodes in the neck will often be swollen. Scratching fingers may also transfer the infection from the scalp to other parts of the child's body, even affecting (rarely) internal organs such as the liver and spleen.

Diagnosis

Severe cases are obvious by simply looking at the child's head. Mild cases will require a closer inspection. If an instrument like a pencil is used to separate the hair, care must be taken not to convey the message that the child is too dirty to touch; the child has no control over his or her problem. A fastidious teacher may be required to act cooler than he or she feels. The examination should be done unobtrusively and privately. If possible, refer the child to the school nurse for diagnostic confirmation—the nurse is, alas, a lice expert.

Teachers may have an aversion to handling a head that houses "crawlers," but there is no reason to fear catching them. Simply wiping the hands with a cloth will ensure safety, since the lice can't jump and the nits are stuck to the hair. Physicians and other health workers have handled hundreds of suspected and infested children without catching lice themselves.

There are several ways to tell the difference between nits and dandruff. A nit should be close to the scalp; a scale of dandruff may be an inch or two away. A nit is stuck to the hair shaft and will not shake off as dandruff will. However, an old nit that has hatched will leave behind a small amount of gelatinous crust that gradually shakes loose.

If there is doubt, recheck the child's head in a day or two, or pluck the suspected hair and look at it under good light.

Treatment

Medications

All medicines used are applied to the hair; none is taken internally. A common prescription medicine is marketed as

"Kwell" by Reed & Carnrick Drug Company. "Rid" is a trademark name also, marketed by Pfizer Drug Company. Both are widely used. There are many other products available. No medicine, prescription or nonprescription, should be used unless it has been recommended by a physician, school nurse, or other health expert. For example, if a child has many sores on his or her scalp and Kwell is applied, it may be absorbed into the bloodstream and cause serious complications.

After one treatment with an effective medication, the lice should all be dead, so the child should be able to attend school the next day.

Mechanical Methods

Simply washing the hair with soap and water every day will completely eliminate head lice in 10 to 14 days. Another method is to use a good-grade hair dryer. Lice are killed (or stunned) at about 120 to 140 degrees Fahrenheit. If the child simply leans over a sink and has his or her hair blown with hot air, this will get rid of almost all of the adult crawlers.

Many products are sold to spray clothes, furniture, and other household items. Save your money. Those sprays are rarely helpful. *Never* use a spray on a child.

The only sure way to eliminate all nits is to soften them with vinegar or similar substance and comb them out with a fine-tooth comb. In a child with thick long hair, this is difficult or impossible.

Action by School Personnel

Should the child, once diagnosed, be sent home immediately? In some schools one-fourth of the class would be sent home if a diligent search were made. If a single diagnosed case stands out like a sore thumb, sending a child home may be considered. In the average public school, however, the answer is an unequivocal **no.** Public health laws in almost all states require exclusion of children with many contagious diseases. Schools, however, recognize degrees of contagiousness and are usually allowed discretion in complying with these statutes. Just as in children with mild colds, sore throats, ringworm, or impetigo—all of which are contagious diseases—if one were to search out and send home all diagnosed cases, too many children would be involved. It's much more practical to send home a note at the end of the school day and save the heavy ammunition (parent conference with the principal or three-day suspensions) for those rare, severe cases in which the parents are completely uncooperative or obstructive. In cases of this nature, the total school management becomes more of an administrative than a medical problem. Not only the principal but often upper-level school administrators, as well as the PTA, could be involved.

SCABIES

Nature of the Condition

Scabies, the original "seven-year itch," is caused by a tiny mite, too small to be seen by the naked eye. In past years it was largely seen in military barracks, orphanages, and other institutions. It was uncommon between the late 1930s and 1960s but is now frequent throughout the United States and is prevalent in many schools. Because it was a rarity for some 30 years, many physicians did not encounter it in their private practice and now may fail to recognize it.

Since the mites live underneath the skin, contagion takes rather prolonged contact, such as children sleeping in the same bed or two children wrestling. A nurse or teacher need never be concerned about touching a child who has scabies—one simply will not get scabies in this manner. All that is required for safety is washing the hands after touching a child with scabies (or lice). Scabies (and lice) are an occupational nuisance rather than a hazard of the teaching profession. School nurses and teachers need to associate and play with children as part of their professional life. On the rare occasions when a teacher does get scabies, it is very easy to cure and should not occasion undue alarm.

Symptoms and Diagnosis

The adult mite burrows beneath the skin of humans and animals. (In dogs and cats, it causes mange.) The mite makes a tiny white bump that itches intensely, particularly at night. As a result of scratching, a scab ½ to 1 millimeter long appears on the skin. The scab tends to be linear rather than round, and this aids in the diagnosis. Another characteristic of scabies is its location on the body. It is commonly found on the backs of the hands, the webs between the fingers, the inner side of the wrist and forearms, and the chest and abdomen. If there are no sores on any of these places, scabies can probably be ruled out. It can also be found on the upper arms and legs, and the neck. It is practically never on the face, on the small of the back between the shoulder blades, on the palms of the hands, or on the soles of the feet. It will often be found on more than one member of the family.

Complications

One of the major complications of scabies is impetigo, an infection of the outer layer of the skin where germs (staphylococcus or streptococcus) normally live. Impetigo is the inevitable result of continued scratching. Once established, it can spread over a large area of the skin surface, become quite severe, and cause more of a problem than the scabies itself. In order to cure this type of scabies, one must first cure the impetigo.

Treatment and Role of the School Nurse

Scabies is easy to cure. Treatment consists of applying one of several different kinds of lotions or ointments, the most effective being lindane lotion, the same one that is used for head lice. The standard method is to apply the lotion from the chin line down to the toes, covering the entire body. The instructions are always outlined in the package insert or can be obtained from the family doctor or school nurse. It is left on for six hours, and then the child is given a bath. The average infestation of scabies will be cured by one application. Some children with severe infestation require two treatments, which should be at least seven days apart. Babies should be clothed so they do not lick their skin. Bed linens and all of the child's clothing should be washed through an ordinary wash cycle in the washing machine. This will eliminate any live scabies, mites, or eggs that might be present. Other methods of treatment, such as benzyl benzoate or sulfur, are effective but rarely used nowadays.

A child with scabies presents no immediate emergency and need not be sent home. By the time the disease is discovered, it has already existed (and has been contagious) for several days or weeks. At the end of the school day, send a note to the parent stating that the child has a contagious skin condition and should not be sent back to school until treated. Remember the sensibilities of the child. Spare him or her any social discomfort by your reaction, and keep your discovery confidential from the other students.

RINGWORM

Nature of the Condition

Ringworm (*tinea*) is a fungus infection of the skin, which is most commonly found in four areas of the body:

1. Scalp—*tinea capitis*
2. Feet—*tinea pedis* (athlete's foot)
3. Genital area—*tinea cruris* (jock itch)
4. Trunk, face, and limbs— *tinea corporis*

Though all four are caused by similar fungi, the appearance and treatment are different depending on the location.

Tinea Capitis

Diagnosis and Role of the School Nurse

The infected scalp typically has small patches of baldness (1 to 3 inches in diameter) that may well be unnoticed under long hair. Boys and girls are equally susceptible, but almost never after puberty. Since the infection affects the hair shaft itself, close inspection reveals tiny, broken-off hairs about 1⁄16 to 1⁄8 inch long. Tinea capitis is often confused with another condition called *alopecia areata,* which also causes round bald spots. In the latter case, the bald spots are absolutely smooth with no broken hairs; the hair falls out by the roots. The differentiation is very important because alopecia areata is completely noncontagious, whereas tinea capitis is one of the most contagious of all diseases and can spread through a school with great rapidity if not controlled. Any suspicious case should be referred to the principal and the school nurse so the child can be sent to the doctor immediately and not allowed back in school until diagnosed and under treatment.

Treatment

The treatment for tinea capitis is always oral medication. Topical ointments will cure ringworm of the body and feet but not of the scalp. The generic name of the oral medicine is griseofulvin, and it only takes a few days of treatment to render the child noncontagious, even though it takes four to ten weeks of treatment for a complete cure. Therefore, the child should not attend school until under treatment for two to five days.

Tinea Pedis

Athlete's foot is much more common in boys than in girls. It responds easily to appropriate lotions or ointments, but unfortunately, it keeps coming back in certain susceptible individuals Many men never completely get rid of it.

Gym teachers are most aware of this condition and usually prepare a solution for the children to step into before going to the showers. While this does no harm, it doesn't really help. Any child with obvious sores on his or her feet should be sent to the school nurse or personal physician for treatment.

Tinea Cruris

This type of ringworm, found in the folds and creases of the body, especially the groin area, is often called jock itch. It is more common in obese individuals, both boys and girls. It is usually quite uncomfortable, itches intensely, and is worse in the summer.

Jock itch is usually caused by various fungi. It is easy to cure, but, like athlete's foot, it often comes back. Cleanliness and certain lotions will cure it very quickly.

Tinea Corporis

Ringworm of the body is very common. It appears on the arm, chest, and abdomen, and a bit more rarely on the face. It starts as a tiny red spot, which slowly grows in a circular fashion, clearing in the center as it enlarges. The edges remain reddish and scaly. No scabs, pus, or crusts are formed as in impetigo. Most children have a single lesion, but on occasion, a child will develop more.

Children often develop small, round, whitish depigmented areas on their cheeks and upper arms. This is definitely not ringworm and is not contagious. Its cause is unknown, but it waxes and wanes without treatment and is completely harmless. If one looks carefully, it is easy to see that the edges of the whitish circular area look the same as the center, thus distinguishing it from ringworm.

Treatment in General

Ringworm of the body, feet, and groin can be treated easily with medicines like tolnaftate (Tinactin), chlortrimazole (Lotrimin), and related compounds. They are not greasy and do not sting the skin or smell bad. Iodine and merthiolate can also be used, but they may sting. The first treatment renders children noncontagious so they can stay in school during treatment until the sores are gone. As stated before, if the scalp is involved, it is necessary to take medicine internally, and it takes two to five days to become noncontagious.

IMPETIGO

Nature of the Condition

Impetigo is a bacterial infection, usually caused by staphylococcus germs, which invades the upper layer of the skin. Probable causes are lowering of body resistance (questionable), hot humid weather (more likely), excess scratching because of lice, insect bites, or scabies (very common). It is more common in children who wash and bathe less frequently.

The most characteristic features of impetigo are the honey-colored and red scabs that cover all or part of each sore. These crusts are easy to pick off or rub off, but usually some bleeding occurs when this is done. The sores may be single and isolated, about ½ inch in diameter, or several may coalesce and form a larger, irregularly shaped sore. Sores are common where children always scratch themselves—on the face, on the fingers, and around the nose. Usually, the palms and soles will be spared.

Since many children have impetigo and it is usually only contagious on direct contact, if there are only a few sores they can be treated and covered with an adhesive bandage, and the child can remain in school. A child with many exposed, visible lesions may have to be sent home.

Treatment

Treatment of impetigo usually requires two steps. First, one must rub or pick off the scab. The germs live under it, and this is where the medicine must be applied. This step hurts a little bit but is necessary. One should soften the scab by soaking and washing the sores with soap and water, then rub hard with gauze or a wash rag. Let the child apply pressure until the small amount of bleeding stops (three to five minutes). One removal is usually sufficient, but if the scab builds up again it may be necessary to repeat the process. Many minor cases can be cured by this treatment alone.

The second step is to apply a little antibacterial ointment (bacitracin is the one most commonly used) and cover with an adhesive bandage if desired. This should be done two to three times a day until the condition is cured. It usually takes only a few days. Other simple antiseptics like merthiolate will also cure small single sores.

It is important to treat impetigo because the sores can continue to spread. In rare cases the germs may find their way into internal organs and form abscesses (boils) in such vital organs as the brain and lungs.

PARONYCHIA OR "FELON"

Nature of the Condition

This is a specialized type of abscess that occurs at the junction of the fingernail and the cuticle. It is almost always associated with nail or cuticle biting or picking.

Symptoms

All symptoms of an abscess are present: pain, redness, swelling, and usually in a day or two, pus. When the pus is still under tension, prior to rupture of the abscess, the tip of the finger may be throbbingly painful. After the abscess ruptures, the pain diminishes and a crust forms.

Occasionally, the abscess circles all around the cuticle—both sides plus the bottom. This is called a "runaround."

Usually, healing is spontaneous, but in some cases infection spreads to the deeper tissues of the finger or hand. This can be most serious and disabling.

Treatment and Action by the School Nurse

At all stages, antibiotic ointment, usually bacitracin, should be applied and the area covered by an adhesive bandage. Sometimes the infection heals without formation of pus.

Prior to formation of free pus, applying hot compresses or soaking the finger in a glass of warm water relieves pain and accelerates healing.

After the formation of pus, it may be necessary to refer the child to the physician so the abscess can be drained by gently inserting a sharp blade between the cuticle and the nail.

If the whole tip of the finger is red and swollen, emergency referral to a physician is mandatory with followup to make sure the parent complies.

Only in rare circumstances should a school nurse attempt drainage with a scalpel blade. If a physician is not available and the school nurse is expected to perform this procedure, there should have been adequate prior instruction and signed standing orders.

BOILS (FURUNCLE)

Nature of the Condition

A furuncle (fyoorunde) is the medical term for a skin abscess or boil. The infection usually starts below the skin and expands. The deeper below the skin that the infection begins, the larger the boil will be when it reaches the surface. Skin abscesses vary in size from one centimeter in diameter to the size of a golf ball.

Causes include insect bites or puncture wounds, like slivers, that deposit germs below the skin surface. These are usually fairly small. Occasionally, germs are deposited under the skin of a child who has a bloodstream infection. These are apt to be larger, the child will be very ill, and will rarely be in school.

Symptoms

The average boil is about ½ to 1 inch in diameter.

1. Initially there will only be pain with minimal swelling and redness at the site of the boil.
2. Within one day the redness and swelling will increase as will the pain.
3. Either that day or the next the center of the boil will begin to show a pale yellow color indicating pus formation.
4. The yellow area enlarges, becomes soft to the touch and may drain spontaneously.
5. In larger abscesses that do not drain properly, the pus gradually gets thick and waxy so that when drainage finally does occur, the pus is apt to come out in one lump. This is known as a *core.*

Treatment

1. Prior to the abscess becoming fluctuant and purulent (soft with pus), warm applications and an antibiotic ointment

such as bacitracin should be applied and covered with a padded protective dressing.
2. When the abscess is at the proper stage, the child should be referred to a doctor to have it opened with a sharp scalpel, not with a needle. Needle openings are too small; they are apt to close before enough pus drains out, and the abscess does not heal properly.
3. Antibiotic ointment should be applied for another day or two until healing is well under way.
4. Don't squeeze the abscess to try to express the core; most abscesses do not have one. In addition to causing needless pain, hard squeezing spreads the infection under the skin and delays healing.

Role of the School Nurse

1. Proper diagnosis and determining appropriate treatment relative to the stage of the abscess is well within the province of the school nurse.
2. Application of warm packs, bacitracin ointment, and protective dressings are appropriate.
3. Rarely should a school nurse lance or otherwise surgically open an abscess with a scalpel or needle. Exactly the same procedures apply as described under Paronychia.
4. Warn others about the dangers of squeezing a boil to express a core.

ACNE

Nature of the Condition

Since about 85 percent of high school children have some degree of acne, it scarcely needs lengthy description. It is usually most severe in girls between ages 14 and 17 and in boys between ages 16 and 19. It usually begins to subside at about age 22 or 23.

It is caused by the action of androgens (male hormones) upon the sebaceous (wax) glands of the skin. The adrenal glands of both boys and girls secrete small amounts of androgen. However, acne is usually worse in boys because the testicles secrete large amounts of androgens during puberty. The sebaceous glands are found in the largest number in the skin of the face, chest, and back. These skin glands secrete sebum or wax, and when they overreact to hormonal stimulation, "whiteheads" or "blackheads" occur. The medical term for these blemishes is *comedo* (pronounced "ká-meh-doe"). A whitehead is a closed comedo and cannot drain out onto the skin surface. It slowly enlarges and bursts out of its capsule under the surrounding skin, gets secondarily infected, and causes a small pimple or abscess (boil). The deeper the original breakout, the larger the boil becomes before it finally ruptures out onto the skin surface or, occasionally, heals without rupturing. In either case, if the abscess is large enough, scarring results. A blackhead is an open comedo that easily drains out onto the skin surface and rarely causes abscesses. The blackened tip is not from dirt or poor hygiene; it is the result of a combination of dead skin cells and skin pigment.

Symptoms

1. *Mild.* The disease is limited to open comedones (blackheads), closed comedones (whiteheads), and occasional small pimples. The lesions are found mainly on the face with a smaller number on the chest and back.

2. *Moderate.* In addition to comedones, pimples, small nodules (hard lumps), and abscesses appear. The shoulders, back, and chest are more involved. The lesions on the face are more numerous. Healing lesions remain red for a long time, but eventually the normal skin color returns.

3. *Severe.* The abscesses are larger, more widespread, and often confluent with several small ones joining to form a large one. There is more reddish discoloration. The larger abscesses heal by scarring and leave a pitted, irregular skin surface.

Emotional Problems

A student with a single pimple is self-conscious. A teenager with moderate to severe acne feels severely socially handicapped. Students do not initiate discussions about these concerns, so they may not know that methods exist to alleviate their problems.

Modern treatment offers many newer and more effective medications that are much more helpful than some of the older remedies. However, successful therapy requires careful and sustained patient cooperation. Support and encouragement by the school nurse can be a key factor in a student's continuing therapy and eventual recovery.

Treatment

1. *Topical therapy (ointments, lotions, and liquids on the skin surface itself).* Most cases can be successfully managed by this method alone. There are innumerable medicines available; some are beneficial, some are of no value, and some are actually dangerous. The older medications usually contain varying combinations of sulfur and salicylic acid. They are usually safe but only minimally effective. The newer medications consist of benzoyl peroxide and vitamin A acid (Retinoic Acid, Tretinoin). These are used singly or in combination and must be applied with careful attention to detail to avoid untoward skin irritation (redness and peeling). These medications should never be used without a physician's supervision. There are many over-the-counter remedies and home remedies for acne. Most are harmless but give little or no help. Some contain mercury and are dangerous; they should never be used.

2. *Oral antibiotics.* The most commonly used oral antibiotic is tetracycline, though others have been used. They are only available when prescribed by a physician and require prolonged usage. They are only used in cases with many pustules and abscesses. Antibiotics can have significant adverse side effects, so careful followup and patient cooperation are necessary. With newer

topical medications, oral antibiotics are not used as much as in the past.

3. *Diet.* For years many foods were thought to cause acne. Sweets, milk, shellfish, fatty foods, ice cream, and chocolate—the arch villain of all—have been implicated. We now know that hot dogs, hamburgers, and candy do not cause acne, nor do they aggravate it. While it is certainly wise for anybody with a known food sensitivity to eliminate that food from their diet, it is now generally recognized by leading skin specialists that no food, even chocolate, causes or worsens acne. However, beliefs about the effects of food persist so strongly that it can be counterproductive to try to dissuade some children. However, if a school nurse encounters a child on any bizarre and obviously unhealthful diet, he or she should definitely intervene through the principal, counselor, parent, or doctor.

4. *Other methods.*

a. Estrogens (female hormones)—for girls over 16 years old with severe acne; potentially serious side effects; occasional good results; careful medical supervision required.

b. Oral retinoids—good results; potentially serious side effects; careful medical supervision required; still experimental.

c. Oral zinc—no proven benefit; potentially serious side effects; to be avoided.

d. Acne surgery—draining of abscesses, comedo removal; helpful if done skillfully.

e. Intralesional therapy—injection of steroids into larger lesions; helpful if done skillfully.

f. Phototherapy—ultraviolet light; value debatable; dangerous if overdone.

g. X-ray—used frequently in past, rarely used today; dangerous.

h. Cryotherapy—freezing of skin with powdered dry-ice slush; requires skilled dermatologist; potential for burn and scar.

i. Scar removal with acid or dermabrasion—for healed, old, severe scars; occasional good results if done skillfully.

j. Oral vitamin A in large doses—of no benefit; usually harmful.

k. Washing of face with cold water, alcohol, or special soaps—psychologically beneficial; rarely harmful; no benefit.

School Relevance and Role of the School Nurse

It is important for principals, coaches, and counselors to be aware of the psychological and emotional implications and for the school nurse to understand them plus the medical or nursing aspects of the disease. The following points should be kept in mind:

1. *Physical education.* Some children, especially girls, have severe acne on the chest, shoulders, and back. They should not be forced to "suit-up" if they strongly object. They are usually willing to express their feelings to a female counselor or school nurse.

2. *Extracurricular activities.* Students with severe acne often need extra encouragement to attend school picnics, pep rallies, dances, and so on. Principals, counselors, and school nurses can play an active role.

3. *Compliance with medication.* Since treatment continues for months or years, and since adolescence is the rebellious period of life, it is common for children with acne not to follow doctors' orders. School nurses, by helping to elevate the students' morale and encouraging and complimenting the students' improved appearance, can motivate improved medication and treatment compliance.

4. *Coordination with physician.* Many acne patients receive physician-prescribed medication. Reports from the school nurse regarding improvement or worsening of the skin or adverse medicine reaction is helpful to the doctor.

5. *Counseling regarding diet and over-the-counter medications.* The school nurse must make sure the student is not using harmful lotions, creams, or liquids. Although the diet should be sensible and well balanced—a properly made hamburger or hot dog can be a complete meal—the school nurse should remain aware that diet plays no role in acne. Parents sometimes think that acne must be outlived, so they do not seek help. The school nurse can open

the door to modern medical therapy through rap sessions or formal classes.

HERPES SIMPLEX

Nature of the Condition

This condition, also called fever blisters, is caused by the *herpes simplex* virus, of which there are two types. (See Figure 2–1.)

Type I is most apt to occur around the lips and nose but can also occur in other facial and body areas. It is extremely common in children; tests show that 70 to 90 percent of adults have had it at some time in their lives.

Type II is most apt to occur in the genital area and is one of the most common sexually transmitted diseases. (See Section 8, Venereal Disease.)

Symptoms

The active sore is the well-known, small fever blister seen on the lip. When the external sore heals, usually in six to ten days, the virus remains latent in the nerve trunks and may be reactivated following excess sunlight, fever, menstruation, and various other forms of physical or emotional stress.

The incubation period for either type of herpes varies from two to twelve days after exposure. Symptoms usually begin with a burning, tingling, or itching sensation at the site where the characteristic sores later appear. Generalized symptoms such as fever, malaise, sore throat, and headache can accompany the initial sores, which generally last no more than three weeks; after healing, no scars remain.

Recurrent sores tend to be less severe than the initial infection and persist for a shorter period of time, about four and a half

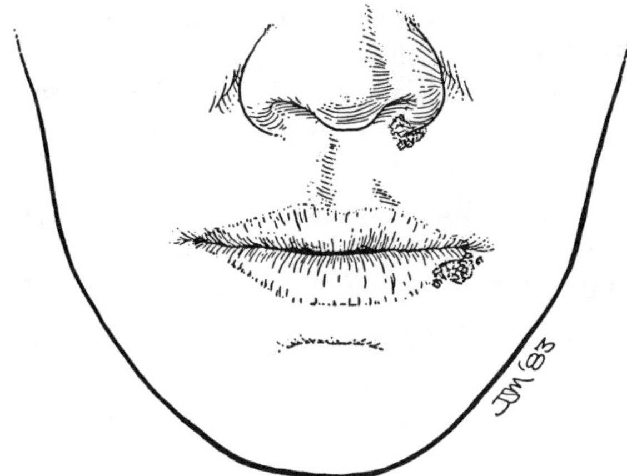

Figure 2–1. Some typical locations of herpes simplex

days. Some children have no recurrent outbreaks while others may experience several recurrences per year.

Modes of Transmission

Both types of herpes are only contagious when the active lesions are present on the skin, *not* during the latent period when the virus is in the nerve trunks.

Type I is usually transmitted by direct contact with infected saliva or the active herpetic lesion itself, while type II is transmitted primarily through sexual contact. As in impetigo, autoinoculation of either type from active lesions on the lips or genitals to other body sites is possible. Since the virus can survive only a short time outside the body, it is unlikely that herpes could be contracted from toilet seats, hot tubs, or other inanimate objects.

Treatment

Currently, there is no medical treatment proven to be completely effective against genital or oral herpes; therefore, medical management should focus on symptomatic relief of pain and discomfort. To enhance healing and prevent secondary infection, the patient should clean the affected area with warm water and soap, and dry it thoroughly.

Various ointments and lotions have been used with some unsubstantiated claims of success; aloe vera and campho-phenique are two of the more common. These are not harmful. Topical application of chloroform and ether have been recommended. They both sting but are not otherwise harmful.

Steroid ointments should not be used. Antibiotic ointments help only if there is secondary bacterial infection.

Prevention

It is important for herpes patients to be careful when handling their lesions to avoid the possibility of transferring the infection to other parts of their bodies. Patients should always wash their hands thoroughly after touching herpes sores. A separate towel should be used to dry an area where lesions are present. Individuals who wear contact lenses should be particularly conscientious so as not to transmit the virus to their eyes. Anyone with active oral herpes lesions showing on their skin should avoid kissing or fondling others, especially newborn infants.

School Relevance and Role of the School Nurse

Many children will come to school with fever blisters (herpes simplex type I). They should not be excluded any more than a child with a common cold, but they should be privately counseled about hand cleanliness and should abstain from close-contact sports such as wrestling.

The nurse's most important function is to allay fears among school personnel and parents. There is a great deal of scare literature available today so people are apt to forget that children have been getting fever blisters for years. It is helpful to collect statements and other educational materials from the local health department.

Both types I and II are spread only by a type of direct contact that is not likely to occur at school. The nurse should advise the principal that disinfecting the classrooms or the bathroom is of no value.

If children with herpes develop multiple lesions around the lips and nose, and especially also on the fingertips, they are likely to have some secondary infection and will respond favorably to the application of antibiotic ointment two or three times a day.

SECTION 3

DISEASES OF THE EARS, NOSE, AND THROAT

This section focuses on the common cold and some of the complications of colds, including middle ear infections, tonsil and adenoid infections, and sinusitis. It also distinguishes between colds and nasal allergy.

THE COMMON COLD

Nature of the Condition and Diagnosis

In medical parlance, a common cold is a viral infection that begins with a runny nose and scratchy throat. Since the lining of the nose joins that of the sinuses, almost everybody with a cold has a certain degree of sinusitis also, even though they may not have any recognizable sinus symptoms. What we call a cold can be caused by some 50 to 60 different types and strains of viruses, each of which causes a slightly different set of symptoms. Some examples are:

1. A one- to three-day runny nose, with no other symptoms, that goes away rapidly and completely.
2. A seven- to fourteen-day runny nose with a slight sore throat and a little cough. There may be a low-grade fever the first day or two. The nasal secretions start clear and runny and gradually thicken and become greenish in color.
3. Same as number 2, with some hoarseness caused by extension of the virus to the larynx (voice box).

With all of the above, the patient may have a little fever the first day or two, a slight feeling of malaise, and some loss of appetite.

4. Similar symptoms but with more fever, ranging from 102 to 104 degrees Fahrenheit in children and 100 to 102 degrees Fahrenheit in adults. This type of cold is the one that causes the most concern and may be associated with some secondary infection requiring specific treatment with antibiotics.

School Relevance and Role of the School Nurse

All colds are much more common in children than in adults. Having a cold usually leaves some immunity to that particular virus, but since there are many others, it takes many years to develop a substantial immunity to the majority of respiratory viruses. Many children seem to catch one cold after another or to have a cold all winter long. Colds are also more severe in children, usually last longer, and cause higher fever and more complications.

Children always come to school with colds. Obviously, they are quite contagious, but it would be folly to try to keep all children with colds at home—the schools would be half-empty. It does the child no harm to attend school provided he or she has no fever and doesn't feel bad.

Treatment

Most colds are overtreated, but usually the treatment is harmless and makes the child more comfortable.

1. Aspirin, Tylenol, and similar types of medications are the most widely used medicines for low-grade fevers and general malaise. They are safe if used in moderation.
2. Nose drops may be necessary; however, a child may experience the negative affects of a rebound reaction which leaves the nose more stopped up than before. Nose drops are advisable only if used in moderation.
3. There are two types of cough medicines. One type is an expectorant, which loosens the secretions and makes it easier to cough. This can relieve dry, hacking coughs which may be very troublesome. A child who cannot rest because of a continuous severe cough may require the second type—a sedative cough medicine. This type usually contains codeine or related substances which can be very helpful if used properly. Because of their nature and mode of action, the sedative cough medicines usually require a prescription and should be used only under a doctor's guidance. If a cough is sedated too much, the retained excess secretions may lead to pneumonia.

The cough is nature's way of clearing undesirable secretions from the respiratory passages and, as such, is beneficial. If the cough does not excessively bother the child, it is not necessary to do anything about it at all. One can be reassured that through coughing, secretions are being forced up out of the lungs and bronchial tubes. Parents as well as teachers often worry because children swallow these secretions. But this is what nature intended; it does no harm whatsoever.

There are dozens of so-called cold remedies on the market today, and many people are convinced that they help—about as many are convinced that they don't help. Most of them contain varying combinations of aspirin, an antihistamine, and an occasional decongestant. My personal philosophy is, "the less medicine the better." Children who are not excessively uncomfortable should be left alone for one or two weeks to get well by themselves. If some of the symptoms (cough or runny nose) cause particular discomfort, follow the recommendations of the doctor or school nurse.

COLDS VS. NASAL ALLERGY

A cold is an acute respiratory infection that begins, runs its course, and ends. It lasts from two or three to fourteen days, depending on the virus. At onset the nasal secretions are thin and clear and gradually get thicker before going away.

Allergies, on the other hand, last a full season, usually spring or fall, or quite commonly all year. The secretions usually stay thin and clear. A cough is less likely to develop. The child usually does not feel bad or have fever.

Unfortunately, many children with nasal allergy get colds more easily and more often than nonallergic children, so they present a mixed picture of a cold implanted on an allergic nasal mucus membrane (inner lining). When this happens, the child who has a runny nose all year will begin to feel bad, perhaps develop a little fever, and often develop a cough. In many cases, even for a physician, it's very difficult to tell one from the other.

Only when the symptoms are very clear-cut or when certain lab tests are available can one be sure.

COMPLICATIONS OF COMMON COLDS

Middle Ear Infections

Symptoms and Diagnosis

A middle ear infection—*otitis media*—is usually a complication of a cold. The younger the child, the greater the incidence of otitis media. By school age, this complication becomes less common than in babies and toddlers. Acute otitis media typically begins with high fever and earache.

Treatment and School Action

This complication always requires treatment by a physician because specific antibiotics are usually needed. Most doctors prescribe treatment for seven to fourteen days. The child usually feels pretty well after the first day or two and may return to school. The antibiotic needs to be continued, however, and it is often given four times a day. This means that on a schedule of 8:00 A.M., 12:00 P.M., 4:00 P.M., and 8:00 P.M., one dose must be given at school. School authorities should always allow this medication to be given by the school nurse or other assigned person because relapses are very common if otitis is not treated diligently enough. Repeated relapses may cause some degree of hearing loss, which proper treatment usually prevents.

Tonsil and Adenoid Infection

Symptoms and Diagnosis

This, too, is usually a complication of a cold, though sometimes the runny nose and cough appear after the fever and sore throat of tonsillitis. The adenoids, located just behind the tonsils, usually get infected at the same time. In addition to the large, red, painful tonsils, the glands (lymph nodes) in the neck also become painful and swollen.

The tonsillitis of a strep throat is caused by a certain streptococcus germ; in this case a throat culture is necessary to identify the germ.

Treatment

Untreated, a strep infection can lead to rheumatic fever with subsequent severe heart damage. Sufficient and correctly chosen antibiotics will prevent this complication.

The Dilemma of Tonsillectomy

Whether or not to remove tonsils is a complicated decision that only an experienced and conscientious physician can properly resolve. This is one of the most commonly overperformed operations, so much so that some insurance companies will pay for a consultant in an attempt to reduce the number. On the other hand, there are certain children for whom tonsillectomy is essential:

1. Recurrent tonsillitis, to the extent that the child fails to grow and thrive and misses school once or twice every month for two to five days despite adequate antibiotics. This child often does exceptionally well after surgery.
2. Frequent middle ear infections. Otitis media is often associated with tonsillitis. Persistent ear infections that do

not respond to medication can result in permanent hearing loss. In these cases, tonsil and/or adenoid removal must be considered.

3. Severe mouth breathing that actually causes the child to be noticeably odd-looking, have some difficulty in swallowing, and snore loudly at night. These children are usually underweight and sickly because of chronic tonsillar infection and are easily susceptible to all infections.
4. Other rare severe conditions, such as peritonsillar abscess.

About 25 to 30 years ago, doctors felt that most children would do better without tonsils and adenoids. As time went by, it was realized that most of this surgery was unnecessary and that there were significant surgical risks and complications. The pendulum swung so far the other way that some children who really needed their tonsils and adenoids removed were denied surgery, especially by younger doctors who were trained in accordance with the newer medical beliefs and who had not had time to see the deleterious effects of long-term tonsillitis. At the present time, there is a good bit of excellent research being carried out to try to define the exact conditions that require surgical removal as opposed to antibiotic treatment. In the meantime, the only safe course is to follow the doctor's advice, but be wary of a too casual suggestion for removal of tonsils and adenoids or a suggestion that the doctor might as well do two or three children in the same family at the same time. In case of doubt, another doctor, preferably an experienced pediatrician, should be consulted. Most responsible doctors do not resent a request for consultation.

Sinusitis

Symptoms

Though the sinuses are always somewhat involved in any cold, in certain cases the cold seems to settle in the sinuses. In these cases, the secretions become thick and greenish-yellow; the cough becomes more prominent and is especially pronounced in the morning. During the night, the secretions collect in the upper air passages after draining from the sinuses into the nose and down the throat. Headache is common, usually over the eyes, but sometimes involving the entire head and increasing in the afternoon. The cough may last a long time, occasionally all winter.

Treatment

Treatment takes a long time. Decongestants, antihistamines, nose drops, and antibiotics are all used for different types of sinusitis. Vaporizers may provide symptomatic relief at night. The long-term outlook is good. Most individuals get completely well, but occasionally, people with nasal allergies develop chronic sinusitis which may last several years.

SECTION 4

EYE PROBLEMS

This section provides a brief glossary of special eye terminology as well as descriptions of specific refractive errors, amblyopia, and conjunctivitis. It emphasizes the importance of checking the child's eyes at an early age.

SCHOOL RELEVANCE

As long as a child is performing well in school and has no complaints, it is usually correctly assumed that the eyes are normal. (See Figure 4–1.) However, as soon as an average child begins to fall behind in schoolwork, one of the first things that occurs to the teacher is to have the eyes (vision) checked, and the eye doctor's report is often difficult to interpret. The best time to check a child's eyes is at age three. Some school nurses and teachers see preschool-age children and should be on the alert for any condition that causes a child to favor one eye over the other.

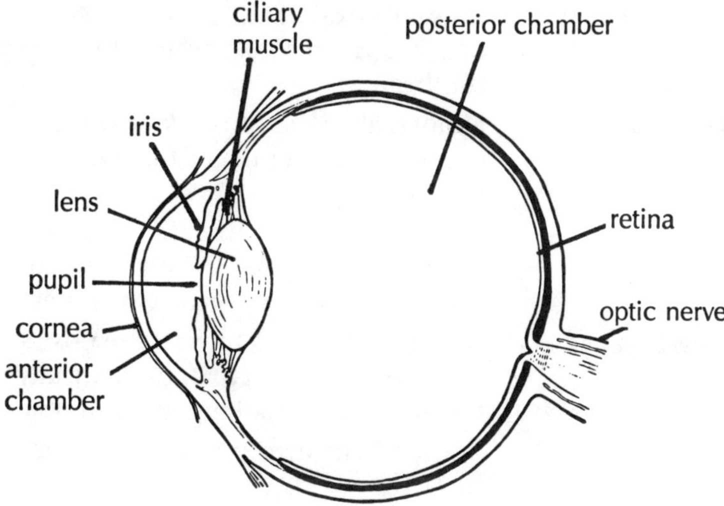

Figure 4–1. Cross-section of the eye.

EYE DICTIONARY

An ophthalmologist, or eye doctor, follows procedures and practices that are highly specialized, more so than almost any other branch of medicine. Therefore, an alphabetical glossary is included here to help understand the unique but necessary vocabulary that describes the abnormalities they see and the procedures they perform. This little "eye dictionary" should help the school nurse understand the ophthalmologist's report and some of the reasoning behind what the doctor suggests.

Accommodation contraction of the ciliary muscle causing the lens to become rounder and therefore thicker. This causes light rays entering the eye to be used for close reading.

Amblyopia blindness of an eye caused by disuse; also called amblyopia exanopsia or *lazy eye*.

Anisometropia a difference in the refractive index of the eyes causing double or blurred vision unless one eye is closed or unless vision in one eye is subconsciously suppressed by the brain.

Astigmatism abnormal shape of the lens (rare) or the cornea (clear center of the eyeball) causing blurred vision.

Conjunctivitis irritation or inflammation of the thin layer of transparent skin covering the eyeball and inner surface of the eyelids.

Convergence both eyes pointing toward the nose simultaneously. This occurs automatically during reading or looking at close objects.

Cross-eye one or both eyes permanently deviating inward.

Diplopia double vision. The child will tend to see two blurred objects rather than one clearly defined.

Divergence both eyes deviating away from the nose simultaneously.

Esophoria one or both eyes deviating toward the nose only on special occasions—if the child is tired, gazing into the distance, or under certain testing conditions.

Esotropia see *cross-eye*.

Exophoria same as *esophoria* but with deviation away from the nose.

Exotropia one or both eyes permanently deviating away from the nose.

Hyperopia farsightedness. The eyeball is shorter than normal, light focuses behind the retina, and vision is blurred.

Myopia nearsightedness. The eyeball is longer than normal, light focuses in front of the retina, and vision is blurred.

Phoria a generic word meaning a tendency for either eye to deviate inward or outward.

Pink eye see *conjunctivitis.*

Strabismus any condition in which the two eyes do not fuse properly and look at the same object at the same time. Also called squint because lack of proper fusion causes *diplopia* so the child closes one eye to see clearly.

Tropia a generic word meaning that either eye actually does deviate inward or outward most or all of the time.

REFRACTIVE ERRORS

There are three kinds of refractive errors. They are hyperopia, myopia, and astigmatism. (See Figure 4–2.)

Hyperopia

Farsightedness—*hyperopia*—can be mild, moderate, or severe. In mild cases, distant vision is normal and only a small amount of accommodation during reading is required to cause the light to

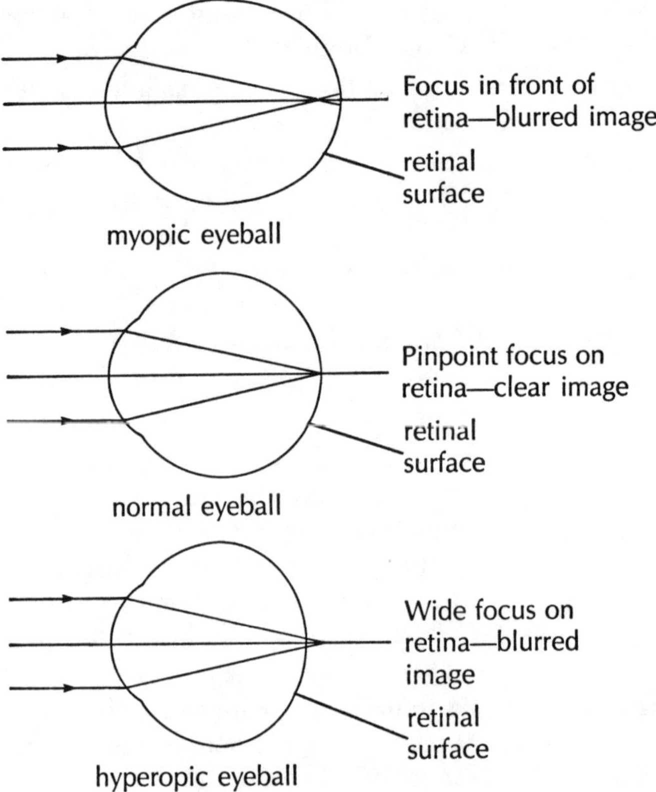

Figure 4–2. Refractive errors

focus exactly on the retina; vision is perfect and glasses are not needed. In moderate cases, distant vision may also be normal, but the child, in order to achieve clear vision while reading close, must accommodate so much that eyestrain develops. This can cause headache, eye pain, fatigue, nausea, and disinclination to read. In severe cases, distant vision is blurred unless strong accommodating efforts are made, and clear vision for reading is impossible. On occasion, reading matter is held close to the nose. Obviously, glasses are necessary for the child with moderate to severe hyperopia.

Myopia

Nearsightedness—*myopia*—exists in varying degrees of severity also, but glasses are always necessary because the light rays already focus in front of the retina and accommodating efforts would merely focus the rays further in front. Myopic children cannot see distant objects clearly but do not know it (never having had normal vision). They are often first discovered during school screening examinations. These children usually hold reading material very close to their noses to be able to see clearly and often squint or frown to see better. This can cause the same symptoms as in hyperopia.

Astigmatism

An irregularly shaped cornea—*astigmatism*—cannot be influenced by accommodation, so glasses are necessary. Holding reading matter close to the eyes, squinting, and frowning are also seen in moderate to severe degrees of astigmatism.

AMBLYOPIA

Nature of the Condition

Visual function is a developmental process of the eye and brain that is not completed until the age of seven years. If vision has not developed by age seven, there is no chance that it will develop later.

Children who do not see equally with both eyes will have double vision. This is so uncomfortable and distracting that these children will rapidly and subconsciously suppress vision in the poorer eye, learn to use only the better eye, and grow up with an eye that is blind because it has never developed a functional connection with the visual centers of the brain. This type of blindness is called *amblyopia,* or lazy eye.

There are two principal abnormalities that cause amblyopia: *strabismus* and *anisometropia.* Strabismus—when the two eyes do not fuse properly to look at an object—is by far the more common of these conditions. Anisometropia is a difference in refractive power in the two eyes. For example, if one eye is hyperopic and the other is myopic, the hyperopic eye will develop amblyopia if not treated. It is said that the overall incidence of anisometropia is 0.5 to 1.0 percent of all children. It is usually discovered in screening programs; a child may see 20/40 with one eye and 20/20 with the other.

Treatment

Once amblyopia is fully established, restoration of vision is impossible. Prevention consists of diagnosing the precursory conditions—strabismus or anisometropia—at a young enough age. If treatment is begun by the age of three, almost all amblyopia can be prevented. With each year of advancing age, the amount of vision remaining becomes less and less, so that by age six or seven permanent blindness has already developed in the amblyopic eye.

From the above discussion, it is easy to see the importance of preschool eye-screening programs. All three-year-old children of average intelligence can be given a reliable vision exam with simple screening tests. Certainly, any child with a squint, abnormal eye movements, or other unusual visual habits should be seen by an eye doctor.

CONJUNCTIVITIS

Nature of the Condition

Conjunctivitis is an inflammation of the thin, transparent outer layer of the eyeball and the inner surface of the eyelids. The inflammation causes redness, tearing, and occasionally formation of pus. Because of the redness, it is commonly called pink eye, and the most common causes are bacteria, viruses, and allergy. The first two are quite contagious. Allergic conjunctivitis is usually associated with nasal allergy and rarely causes any pus in the inner corner of the eye; this can be helpful in differentiating contagious from noncontagious varieties.

Treatment

Bacterial conjunctivitis is the cause of about 55 to 65 percent of cases of pink eye. Treatment usually consists of antibiotic eye drops or ointments, and most cases heal very quickly. However, if the infectious conjunctivitis is caused by a virus, antibiotic drops will not help. Therefore, some children with mild pink eye will be told by their physician that no treatment is necessary, and the condition will go away by itself in a few days.

Allergic conjunctivitis can be relieved, not cured, by certain nonantibiotic eye drops.

Parents should be warned not to use over-the-counter medications containing mercury; some children are highly sensitive and can develop serious reactions to it.

Role of the School Nurse

Each child with pink eye should be evaluated by the school nurse. If the pink eye appears infectious, it should be referred to a physician; if allergic, it can be observed for a day or two to see if it goes away. If no medication is prescribed, the child should be observed daily; if the condition worsens, the doctor or parent should be notified.

If public health laws mandate that children with pink eye stay home, then the school nurse has no option. However, although most pink eye is contagious, it is not always medically necessary to exclude children from school for more than a day. Common colds are also contagious, and we do not insist that children with colds stay home. This is one of the difficult decisions school nurses must face.

ADEQUATE LIGHTING

How much light (usually measured in candlepower or lumens) should be present for adequate reading and writing? There is much literature on this subject, but most of it is less than scientific. The amount of light necessary for school children to perform academic tasks comfortably varies, but 50 lumens per square foot of reading surface is often considered optimal. A 60-watt incandescent bulb emits about 850 to 900 lumens of light. A 60-watt (four foot) fluorescent bar emits about 3300 to 4300 lumens. However, many children do quite well studying under 20 to 30 lumens per square foot for long periods. For shorter periods even 10 lumens reduces efficiency only 7 percent.

It is often stated that children reading with inadequately directed light or in dim light will develop eye strain. In actuality, children and adults with normal eyes, with or without glasses, can read quite comfortably in a wide range of candlepower and with light coming from a variety of sources. In general, if a teacher with normal eyes can read comfortably, he or she can rest assured that the students can also. In addition, there are no long- or short-range ill effects on the eyes if one reads for short periods with less than adequate lighting.

Recently there have been concerns about the types of light bulbs used. In the classroom, old-fashioned incandescent bulbs and both types of fluorescent bar bulbs—cool white and daylight—have proved to have no adverse effect on children. The two newer lights—sodium vapor which casts a yellowish light and mercury vapor which casts a bluish light—have been reported to cause stomach aches, headaches, nervousness, and other vague symptoms in some children. Therefore, they should be used only in open playgrounds and not in enclosed classrooms.

SECTION 5

DISEASES OF THE LUNGS

This section covers five diseases of the lungs: asthma, bronchitis, pneumonia, tuberculosis, and pleurisy. It also discusses the controversial matter of asthmatic children's participation in sports and the involvement of the physician in the asthmatic child's school program.

ASTHMA

Nature of the Condition

Asthma is an allergic disease of the lungs that causes constriction of the smaller bronchioles (small air passages). The typical attack causes moderate to severe difficulty in breathing. There is always some associated wheezing even though it may not be audible to the unaided ear. The children always experience some degree of distress and anxiety—the more severe the attack, the more anxious and worried they are.

In many cases, the allergic asthmatic attack is accompanied by an infection in the respiratory tract. When this occurs, the child has significant fever and may need antibiotics in addition to asthma medicine.

School Relevance

Asthma is one of the most common serious illnesses of the school-age child. It is not serious in the sense of being life-threatening, but it does in many cases affect a child's entire life style. Children with moderately severe asthma miss school often, must visit the doctor frequently, make many trips to hospital emergency rooms, and have probably been hospitalized several times. They take a lot of medicine and get many shots. Also, they are socially limited. They come to be known as sickly and in time think of themselves that way. With all of this, it is easy to see why the disease has an effect far beyond the actual wheezing episode. Fortunately, most children "outgrow" their asthma. Attacks occur very frequently in preschool and elementary school children, but by middle school years they usually diminish in frequency and intensity.

Physical Education and Asthma

Participation in sports is controversial. Until eight to ten years ago, doctors felt that children with asthma should not be overly active because running and playing usually exaggerate the coughing and wheezing. Children with a condition called *exercise-induced asthma* do not wheeze until they do something that makes them breathe fast. Hard laughing and running will bring on an attack.

Doctors, as well as parents, prefer that asthmatic children avoid activities known to bring on attacks. An overzealous physical education teacher may insist that all children exercise every day. Lest anybody point the finger at gym teachers for being cruel and heartless, it must be said that many doctors will write an excuse from gym for long periods (sometimes all year) on very flimsy grounds. In any case, teachers should know that some asthmatic children should limit exercise and for a certain period in their lives must forego the pleasures and benefits of active competitive sports. However, this does not in any way mean that asthma should preclude total participation in all sports. Relatively quieter sports such as archery or golf are salutary and maintain body tone without increasing the respiratory rate.

Most children with asthma are perfectly normal between attacks and should be allowed to exercise to the full limits of their tolerance. With the recent increased emphasis on physical fitness, jogging, and so on, it is current practice to recommend graded exercise for asthmatic children to enhance general body strength and muscle tone in the hope that they will get fewer attacks, be able to better withstand the attacks they do get, and generally lead a more happy and productive life. While this has not yet been proven, it seems reasonable.

Many children with asthma are overprotected by parents and doctors to the point that they themselves become convinced that any exercise will bring on an attack. Because of the emotional aspects of asthma, they are often correct. This type of child would probably be helped by graded and carefully monitored physical exercise. Unfortunately, there are very few public schools in the United States that employ special adaptive physical education teachers to develop special programs for handicapped children. If encouraged to exercise without guidance, children will typically overexert themselves past their point of tolerance. Many adult males do the same thing when they enter an exercise program.

Physician Involvement

The child with asthma often ends up in the center of a triangle with parents at one corner, doctor at the other, and physical education teacher at the third. All too often they are not working cooperatively. The parents tend to be overprotective, the physical education teacher overdemanding, and the doctor too casual and unable (or unwilling) to understand the social and psychological implications of the school problem. To avoid such a situation, the doctor, parents, and physical education teacher—each respecting and understanding the other—should confer, discuss the situation rationally, and agree on a plan for the year. If this requires more time than they can give, a three-way telephone conference is a useful substitute. This problem usually arises in sixth or seventh grade, and by that time the methods of coping and the relationship among the child, the parents, and the doctor have been well established. If a child has a note from the doctor saying that he or she should be excused from physical education for the whole year because of asthma, teachers should not be too insistent on physical education participation. Refer the problem to the principal to deal with as an administrative matter. It is a mistake to equate physical fitness with total health. One or two years without physical education are not crucial in a child's lifetime, and most children outgrow their asthma (or most of it) by high school.

Treatment

Certain health professionals teach young children to participate in managing their own asthma. How successful this will be remains to be seen. This approach is described in an excellent book by Parcel, Tiernan, Nader, and Weiner entitled *Teaching Myself about Asthma* (Saint Louis: C.V. Mosby, 1979). This book should be helpful for teachers as well as children in understanding the nature and management of asthma.

Each child with asthma requires a highly individualized form of treatment. Antibiotics, broncho-dilators, allergy shots, respiratory therapy, and so on, are all used in varying degrees. Mild cases are often cared for by family physicians, but moderate to severe forms usually require the skills of pediatricians and allergists.

BRONCHITIS

Nature of the Condition and Symptoms

Bronchitis is an infection of the bronchial tubes which carry the air down to the air sacs in the lungs where oxygen is absorbed into the bloodstream. This condition can follow a cold, and though the children usually feel well and have no fever, a troublesome cough persists for several weeks after the cold goes away. On a winter walk through the school halls it sometimes sounds like a small herd of walruses. The cough usually starts out "tight"—dry, hacking, and nonproductive of sputum. Later it gets looser, wetter, more productive, and less frequent. It often takes four to six weeks to go away. In some children with allergic bronchitis, the cough can last all winter.

Treatment and School Relevance

The only medicines available for this condition are cough medicines. They are not very effective in controlling the cough unless one gives relatively large doses of sedative cough medicines, and this can suppress the cough so much that dangerous amounts of secretions are retained in the lungs. The cough is almost always made worse by physical exertion, so it may help to limit physical education and/or recess. During the time when the cough is severe, though it sounds horrible, it is not very contagious. Whether or not children should stay home depends on how much the cough bothers the child and others.

PNEUMONIA

Nature of the Condition

Pneumonia is an infection of the air sacs of the lungs. In the past several years, many physicians have been using the word *pneumonitis* instead of pneumonia. Though the two words mean the same thing, it has become common practice to use pneumonitis when one means a small area of infection with minimal symptoms, and pneumonia for larger areas of infection with more severe symptoms.

Normal lungs are soft and spongy since they are filled with air. When a child develops pneumonia, the involved portion of the lung becomes very dense and consolidated.

The lungs are divided into separate portions called lobes—two on the left and three on the right. Infection of an entire lobe is called lobar pneumonia. When the infection involves smaller patches in one or several places simultaneously, it is called bronchopneumonia.

There are many different kinds of pneumonias. Acute lobar pneumonia with a very high fever can occur very suddenly and is still a formidable cause of death in many parts of the world. However, with proper diagnosis and treatment, it is usually one of the easiest diseases to cure. On the other hand, bronchopneumonia caused by certain types of viruses can be so mild that the child has only a mild cough and a very low-grade fever and is hardly sick. It is these very mild types that are often referred to as *walking pneumonia*.

Symptoms

School nurses have reason to suspect pneumonia when the following symptoms are present:

1. *Cough.* Almost all children with pneumonia have some type of cough, the most common being a relatively small loose cough that is not overly troublesome.
2. *Fever.* High fever is present in most children but occasionally it will be low.
3. *Lassitude, loss of appetite, drowsiness, and general malaise.* These latter symptoms, of course, are common to almost all children's illnesses.

School Relevance and Role of the School Nurse

The child with frank pneumonia is usually quite sick and therefore will not be in school. Teachers and nurses, however, will see many children with a cough who may have a temperature of 100 to 100.6 orally. When these symptoms are combined with those listed in the third group above, it is wise to refer the child to a doctor, especially if, after a day or two, the child does not run and play as usual. Since pneumonia presents such a highly variable set of symptoms, it is not wise for a teacher, principal, or parent to wait too long before having the child examined.

While a few specific varieties of pneumonia are contagious, the types that are most often seen in school are not. Most pneumonia is caused by germs or viruses that are present in healthy children, and the children who actually develop disease in their lungs do so because of individual susceptibility—not by catching it from another child who may come to school with pneumonia.

Treatment

All children with pneumonia need a certain amount of rest. Almost all of them need antibiotics. The treatment should always be managed by a physician.

TUBERCULOSIS

Nature of the Condition

There are two types of *tuberculosis:* primary, usually occurring in childhood, and secondary, usually occurring in adults. The primary type represents the body's first encounter with the tuberculosis germ (*tubercle bacillus*). The infection localizes in the lymph nodes near the center of the lungs and in most cases is self-cured by normal body resistance. While there are no outwardly visible traces, an x-ray sometimes shows permanent evidence of healed tuberculosis. The incidence of primary tuberculosis is diminishing.

Primary tuberculosis triggers a change in the body's immune reaction mechanism. The entire body, including the skin, becomes allergic to the tubercle bacillus for many years thereafter. Therefore, if a tuberculin skin test is performed, it causes a typical reddish reaction. If the same skin test is performed on a person who has never had tuberculosis, it will cause no reaction. When a child first shows a positive skin test, it is necessary that he or she have a chest x-ray to make sure that the disease is not in its active stage. While most primary tuberculosis is mild and cures itself, an unusual case may require extensive treatment.

Treatment

Streptomycin, discovered in the mid-1940s, was the first medicine available to treat tuberculosis. Now it is reserved for certain rare and severe types. Most cases can be cured with several other oral medications.

As a precautionary standard practice, all children with a positive skin test are treated for one year, usually with INH (isonicotinic acid hydrazide) alone. This prevents any possibility of a severe and sometimes fatal complication that may follow childhood tuberculosis.

Contagiousness

Adult tuberculosis is contagious; the childhood type is not at all contagious. This paradox arises from the fact that children with childhood tuberculosis do not cough up tuberculosis germs. Childhood or primary tuberculosis settles in a part of the lung near the center and does not irritate the bronchial tubes; therefore, there is no cough to spread the germs into the air. Older children or teenagers, of course, may develop the adult type (also called secondary tuberculosis). If they do, they cough and are just as contagious as adults. Obviously, a doctor's advice is necessary to determine whether any individual child with tuberculosis is contagious or not.

School Attendance

Many years ago, children with diagnosed tuberculosis had to miss months or even a whole year of school. Today, medication is so effective that after an initial two- to five-day period of treatment, children may attend school without harm to themselves or others. Treatment usually continues for at least a year.

PLEURISY

Pleurisy, an infection of the thin outer skin of the lungs, can occur as an infrequent complication of pneumonia or tuberculosis. Pleurisy causes more severe chest pain, higher fever, and occasionally an outpouring of fluid between the lung and the chest wall called *pleural effusion.* Intensive treatment is required.

Pleurisy caused by some of the other viruses can also be present independent of pneumonia. This type of pleurisy almost never causes effusion though it can cause a moderately severe, constricting type of pain in the chest. Therefore, it has come to be known as the grippe or devil's grippe. It is self-limiting, going away in seven to fourteen days, and requires no antibiotic treatment.

SECTION 6

DISEASES OF THE HEART

This section covers the nature, symptoms, diagnosis, school relevance, and treatment of four types of heart conditions: acquired heart disease, rheumatic fever, congenital heart disease, and heart murmurs. It stresses special caution in detecting heart murmurs since many children possess soft and quiet functional murmurs that have no significance at all.

ACQUIRED HEART DISEASE

Nature of the Condition

This type of heart disease can occur in children of school age. It may be caused by viruses, bacteria, or, rarely, fungi, and it can attack a perfectly healthy child. It may occur by itself, but most often it occurs as a complication of another primary disease. This primary disease may be serious, such as diphtheria, or it may be a mild virus infection.

The heart has three distinct layers: outer, middle, and inner. Infection of the outer layer, or pericardium, is called *pericarditis.* In the middle, or myocardium, it is called *myocarditis,* and in the inner layer, or endocardium, it is called *endocarditis.*

Symptoms and Diagnosis

All acquired heart disease makes children seriously ill with fever and prostration. They rarely want to get out of bed. The heart rate is usually quite rapid, even faster than one sees with the same amount of fever from other disease. The heart may also beat irregularly.

School Relevance and Treatment

All acquired heart disease of acute onset as described above makes children so sick that it is unlikely they will be in school. However, if a child appears sicker than the degree of fever would indicate, especially if the heart rate is very rapid and/or irregular, he or she should be allowed to rest in the clinic until the parents can pick him or her up. Definitive treatment will depend on the exact diagnosis and must always be carried out by the child's physician.

RHEUMATIC FEVER

Nature of the Condition

This is a special type of acquired heart disease that is caused by a particular body sensitivity to the same streptococcus germ that causes scarlet fever and strep throat. After complete recovery from rheumatic fever, a few children are left with heart valves in a damaged condition. Of the four heart valves, the mitral valve is the one most commonly involved. After several years, this valvular damage causes symptoms that can gradually become severe.

Symptoms

The early symptoms of chronic rheumatic heart disease are mild shortness of breath, especially on exertion, occasional mild chest pain, and occasionally slight blue color around the lips. Eventually, the heart enlarges a great deal, it weakens, and actual heart failure ensues. It takes several years after the initial attack for significant valvular damage to occur. While most cases of valvular disease do not cause noticeable symptoms until young adult life, occasionally symptoms appear in children of secondary school age.

School Relevance

Some children with chronic rheumatic carditis may be in school. If so, they may have a note from their doctor asking for some restriction of physical activity. If this should occur, the teacher should readily accede to the doctor's request.

This is a rare disease, especially in southern climates with milder winters. Better treatment of early streptococcus infections has helped to cause this welcome decline in the incidence of rheumatic heart disease.

CONGENITAL HEART DISEASE

Nature of the Condition

Congenital heart disease is present when the child is born and can be inherited or caused by disease or distress of the embryo during its development. It is usually characterized by a

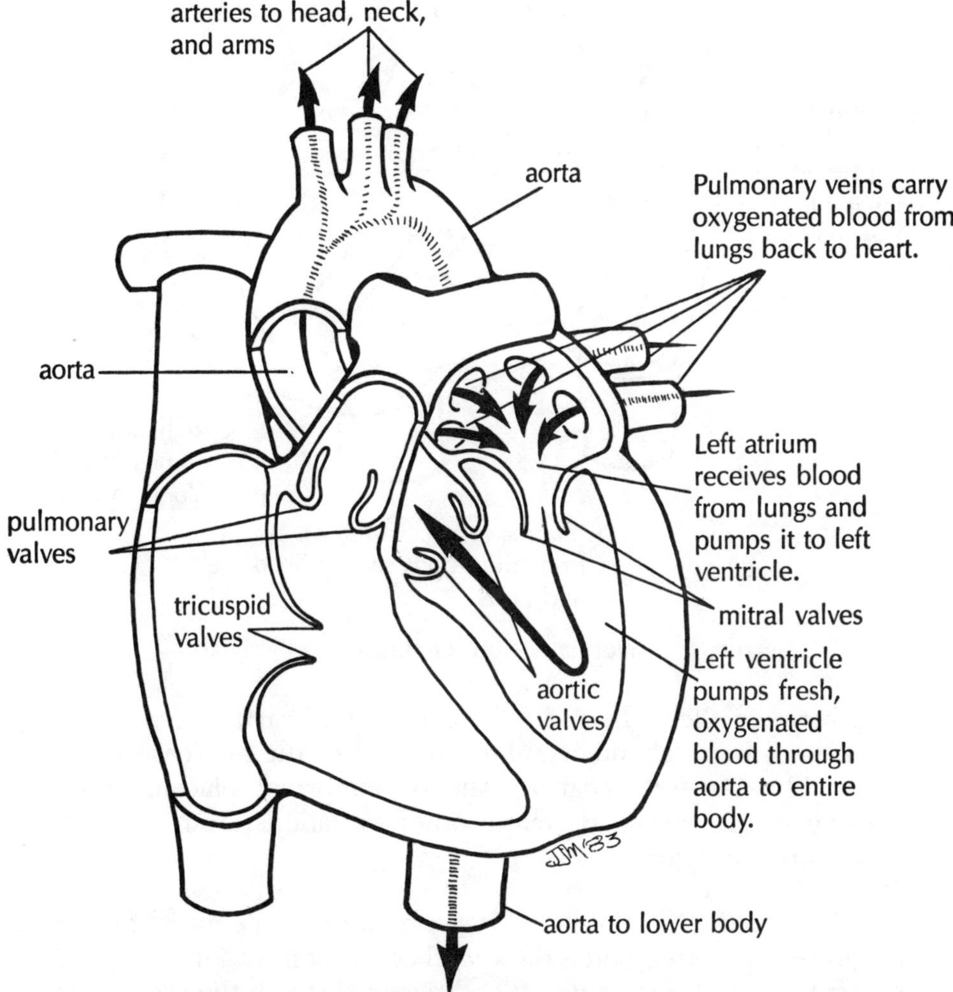

Figure 6–1. Normal arterial circulation in the heart

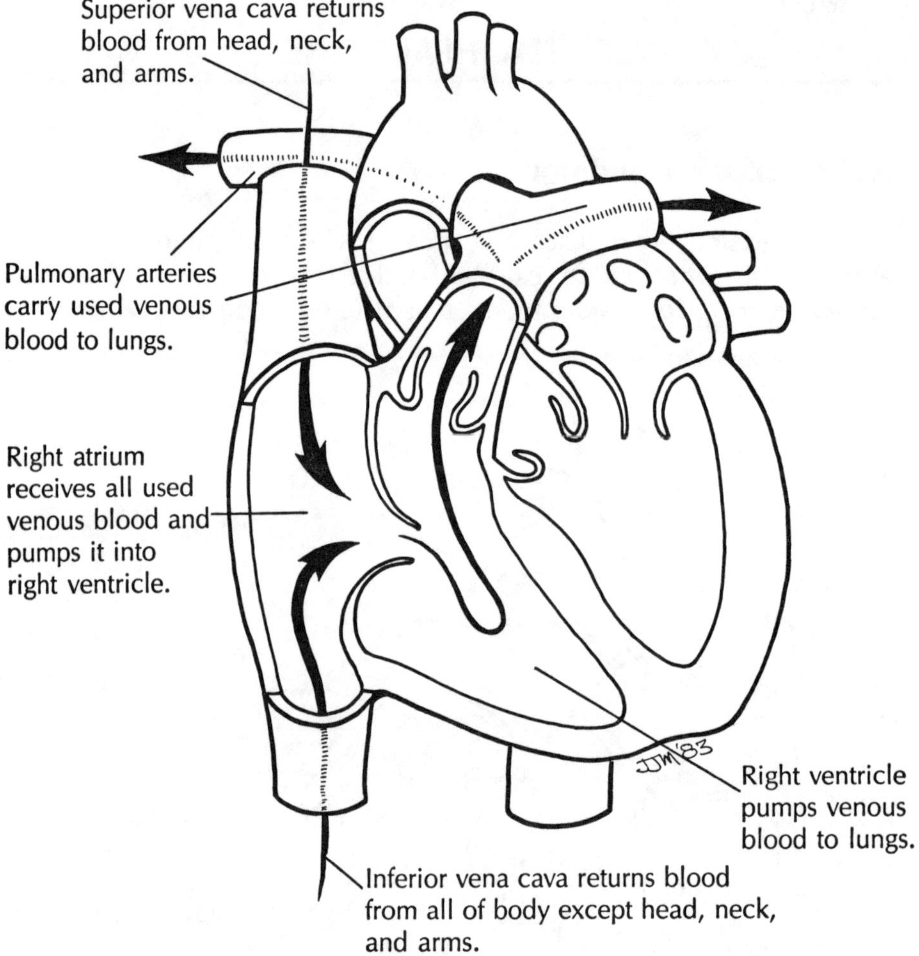

Figure 6–2. Normal venous circulation in the heart

hole between the right and left sides of the heart, an abnormal number of heart chambers, abnormalities of the heart valves or major blood vessels near the heart, abnormal placement or twisting of the heart, or many other variations from normal. There are two types:

1. *Cyanotic.* Arterial blood has a high oxygen content and is bright red; venous blood is dark red because it has a lower oxygen content. As dark red venous blood passes through the lungs, it is reoxygenated and pumped out through the arteries to the body.

In most cases of cyanotic congenital heart disease, venous blood enters into, mixes with, and darkens the arterial blood. This causes cyanosis, a purplish-blue coloration especially seen through the fingernails and on the lips.

2. *Noncyanotic.* When arterial blood is pumped into the veins, the mixture goes through the lungs to become oxygenated again before going back out to the body, so it becomes bright red again and the skin color is normal.

Symptoms

Cyanotic Type

1. Cyanotic children exhibit a bluish tinge around the lips and fingertips. After several years the fingertips become swollen. This is called *clubbing.*
2. All of the tissues receive a poor oxygen supply, impairing body growth. Resistance to infection is low; the child is sickly and frequently absent from school.
3. Breathing is deeper and faster to get sufficient oxygen. Very little exercise is tolerated, requiring frequent rest. Chronic shortness of breath makes speaking difficult.
4. The brain receives less oxygen, which impairs cerebral processes in many subtle ways. Many of these children have learning problems.

The extent of the symptoms depends on the amount of the oxygen deficit. Other factors that influence the severity of the symptoms are the size of the heart, the regularity of the heartbeat, and the blood pressure.

Noncyanotic Type

In many cases this causes no symptoms at all, at least in childhood. As the child grows older, the heart gets abnormally large because of the extra workload, having to pump a larger-than-normal volume of blood. The enlarged heart is a weak heart and eventually decompensates (fails). When this happens, the child begins to show many of the same symptoms as the child with cyanotic heart disease.

HEART MURMURS

Most children with congenital heart disease will have significant murmurs that can be heard with a stethoscope by a physician or a school nurse with proper training and experience. However, caution is necessary.

Many children have very soft, quiet heart murmurs that are called functional. These murmurs are very common—about 50 percent of children have them. They come and go from day to day. *They have absolutely no significance whatsoever. They are normal.*

Functional murmurs are often heard in school screening programs. If proper rechecking is not done, these children, who need not and should not go to a doctor at all, are referred to a doctor. Some of them are subjected to a great many unnecessary tests, some of which may be risky in and of themselves. Further, the children come to think of themselves as having an abnormal heart and develop an unhealthy attitude toward their own physical capabilities.

A pediatric cardiologist can sort out some of these murmurs simply by listening to them, thus sparing the child any tests at all, even a simple x-ray of the chest. Most of the time, only a chest x-ray and electrocardiogram will be necessary—both entirely harmless and painless. Only about 10 to 15 percent of cases referred to most specialists will require invasive techniques (intravenous dye injection or inserting a long flexible tube through a vein into the heart), and this number is gradually getting smaller as a result of the development of new techniques. These latter tests require hospitalization and carry some small risk, though in the presence of serious congenital heart disease they are invaluable and necessary.

Treatment

In both types of heart disease in children of school age—cyanotic and noncyanotic—treatment consists of surgical repair of the abnormality. Not all congenital cardiac abnormalities can be repaired. Some are so severe and complicated that complete cure by surgery is impossible. In these cases, palliative procedures often can be performed that give partial relief. In most cases, however, surgical cure is possible.

A word of caution is advisable. The modern-day diagnosis and surgical correction of congenital heart disease are extremely complicated and should be done only by a pediatric cardiologist and skilled cardiac surgeon. If their services are not available locally, the child should be taken to a larger medical center.

School Relevance

Many children with congenital heart disease attend school every day. Most are in mainstream regular classes. Some have had operations to correct their heart defects, and some have not.

Children who visit a doctor for regular checkups are fortunate because this type of heart problem is usually diagnosed with a stethoscope. A murmur, by its sound and location, can guide the cardiologist to perform the kinds of tests that lead to an exact diagnosis. There are many children, however, especially in the so-called inner-city schools, who rarely if ever visit a doctor. They may go for years with their hearts slowly enlarging and gradually becoming more and more damaged. By the time they start having symptoms, it is usually too late to effect a complete cure.

Role of the School Nurse

Most children with congenital heart disease will be under a physician's care. The school nurse should maintain contact with the doctor's office for any special instructions that may be necessary. The nurse should also act as an intermediary between the educational and medical personnel to make sure the efforts of both are coordinated for the child's welfare. This will be especially true in two instances:

1. *Special education.* If the child is not performing at academic potential, this may be because of general weakness or lack of oxygen to the brain. The school nurse may contribute to the development of an individual educational plan.

2. *Restriction of physical activity.* Almost all children with congenital heart disease can be allowed to regulate their own activity; they will stop when tired. However, the school nurse may need to reinforce teachers' efforts to keep some overeager children from exceeding their capabilities.

SECTION 7

DISEASES OF THE BRAIN

This section covers the condition, symptoms, school relevance, and treatment of epilepsy, rabies, cerebral palsy, developmental dyspraxia, and progressive diseases of the brain such as multiple sclerosis. Included is a chart to help distinguish between real and pseudo epileptic seizures.

EPILEPSY

Nature of the Condition

Epilepsy is one of the medical conditions that almost every teacher and school nurse will have to deal with, in one way or another, several times during a school career. It is a relatively common affliction and is seen much more often in children than adults. For unknown reasons, most children outgrow their epilepsy during their teens. Also, treatment is effective in most cases, and this too can shorten the natural course of a disease which, untreated, can have a serious potential.

Each individual epileptic attack or seizure is extremely frightening to school personnel, especially the typical grand mal seizure or major convulsion. However, children are unlikely to harm themselves during a seizure. Contrary to popular belief, epileptics rarely bite their tongues and many authorities maintain it is not necessary to insert something between the teeth, though some still recommend insertion of a padded stick. The major cause of concern is possible brain damage from repeated, uncontrolled convulsions. During a convulsion, the patient stops breathing for a brief period of time and the entire body is deprived of oxygen. The brain—the organ most sensitive to lack of oxygen—suffers most, and on occasion a certain number of brain cells die. Once a brain cell dies, it never regenerates, and eventually, with the death of enough cells, brain damage occurs and learning disability or mental retardation may occur. It is well known that many kinds of brain damage are more common in epileptics, and this is one of the reasons.

Most epileptics are perfectly normal in all respects other than their occasional seizures. Those who have severe and frequent attacks, however, either because of poor compliance with medical treatment or because their disease is so severe, eventually develop some degree of noticeable brain damage. Also, since pathology in one part of the brain is often associated with abnormalities in other parts, even well-controlled epileptics have a higher incidence of subtle learning and behavior problems as well as a higher incidence of frank intellectual retardation.

Symptoms and School Relevance

Epilepsy is often classified by the nature of the seizure, and different types often respond best to different medications. There are many types but only four will be discussed here. The others are rare or only seen in infancy.

Grand Mal Seizures

This is a typical hard-shaking convulsion. It is liable to occur at any time, but some authorities feel it is more likely to occur when the child is at rest than when he or she is engaged in some sort of mental or physical activity. It sometimes begins with an aura—the child will see a light or halo or experience an unusual feeling. At this time, the child is still conscious and will appear frightened. Almost immediately, however, the convulsion will begin with a sudden, rigid stiffening of the entire body—so stiff and so strong that the back is arched, and if the child were able to be balanced on his or her back only the heels and head would touch the ground. The instant this begins, consciousness is lost and the child falls to the ground. This is called the tonic phase of the convulsion, during which all of the muscles of the body are held extremely tight. The jaw is tightly clenched and no effort should be made to open it. Broken teeth (and lawsuits) have resulted from overzealous efforts. This lasts 20 to 40 seconds and leads into the clonic phase. During this second phase, the true shaking convulsion begins because of intermittent contractions of body muscles. It is during this period that one may gently insert a padded stick between the teeth. The third stage is one of deep sleep and lasts 5 to 30 minutes. Following this stage, the child awakens and, except for muscle soreness, is as normal as before.

What has been described here is a typical or average convulsion, though any one convulsion is apt to be a little bit different—longer or shorter, more or less severe. Sometimes, in a mild attack, there is no period of deep sleep. Sometimes the seizures are limited to one side of the body or only one extremity with no loss of consciousness. These are called Jacksonian seizures.

Petit Mal Seizures

These are also called *absence spells*. They are extremely brief episodes, lasting one to three seconds, during which the child loses consciousness but does not lose body tone and usually does not fall down. If the child is holding something, a pencil or glass, he or she is apt to drop it. During this brief period the child is completely out of contact. When the episode is over, the child will resume activity, completely unaware that anything has happened.

The child with petit mal epilepsy often has 20 to 40 episodes a day. As with grand mal seizures, there usually are some variations in the appearance of the seizures. There may be occasional twitching of the facial or arm muscles. Sometimes an attack can last five to ten seconds. Many are so brief that nobody ever knows they have occurred. Contrary to grand mal seizures, this type of epilepsy does not cause brain damage.

Teachers often wonder if certain children have petit mal epilepsy because they lack attention or stare out of the window or do not hear something that was said, and they will refer the child to a physician. Many doctors have been upset about this because, even though they feel sure from the described symptoms that the child does not have epilepsy, once the suspicion has been raised they are obligated to proceed with some fairly expensive tests (EEG, x-ray, etc.), which most of the time show normal results. However, classroom experience shows that teachers do have some reason to wonder about some children.

It is very difficult to give good guidelines about just which episode may be a petit mal attack and which is a simple wandering of attention. One important factor is frequency of occurrence. If the spell only occurs occasionally, not even every day, it is more likely to be just lack of attention. Also, if the teacher looks closely, the pupils of the eyes will always be enlarged during a petit mal seizure and they will not constrict even if a bright light is shined into them. If the child is touched during an episode, he or she will not notice it. If the child drops whatever he or she may be holding, this is also suggestive evidence.

In summary, if the teacher or school nurse is not sure and if the attacks are infrequent, it is much better to wait and watch until more definitive signs appear. This course of action will result in much less anxiety and less needless expense for the family.

Psychomotor Epilepsy

This is a rare type of epilepsy in which an attack causes the patient to engage suddenly in a spurt of coordinated muscular activity that may appear to be under voluntary control.

> The seizures are characteristically of brief duration, lasting from a minute to 5 to 10 minutes. Consciousness is often impaired but rarely completely lost. The most common motor symptoms are drawing or jerking of the mouth and face ... Aphasia or dysphasia may be present ... The eyes may stare in a searching manner. There may be tonic posturing or a desire to urinate. Coordinated but inappropriate movements may be performed repeatedly in a stereotyped manner (automatism), common examples being clutching, fumbling, kicking, walking or running in circles, swallowing, smacking, chewing, licking, and spitting. Pill-rolling,...[twisting hand or arm movements,] or flinging movements [of the arms] are less common. Inhibitory seizures with loss of tone (limpness) or arrest of motion (freezing) may occur. Affective expressions such as laughing or crying are not unusual.... When the attack is over, there may or may not be ... sluggishness or sleep. Amnesia of the attack is the rule. (From Barnett, *Pediatrics,* 15th Ed. used with permission from Appleton-Century-Crofts.)

Epileptic Equivalents

Episodic vomiting, diarrhea, dizziness, vertigo, and even episodes of seeming insanity have been blamed on epilepsy. Needless to say, these common symptoms are rarely caused by epilepsy. A pediatrician can easily rule out epilepsy in more than 99 percent of cases of this nature. Diagnosis of that one remaining percent is difficult even for skillful neurologists using all of the diagnostic tools at their command.

Diagnosis

Certain factors are common to all forms of epilepsy:

1. *Sudden onset and relatively rapid termination.* Epilepsy usually begins when least expected, for no apparent reason, runs its course, and stops.

2. *Loss of memory.* This occurs in all forms of epilepsy except the epileptic equivalents. Remembrance of the episode is so unusual in epilepsy that it makes some neurologists skeptical that there is actually a condition called epileptic equivalents. Typically, when epileptic attacks are over, patients awaken in a dazed state wondering what happened to them. If they have suffered many attacks, they will be able to guess what happened but will not remember it.

3. *Repeated attacks.* It is very rare for a person with epilepsy to have a single attack. Occasionally a child will be diagnosed and treated after the first attack and never have another, but this is quite rare.

When all three of the above factors are present, the diagnosis is easier to make. Physicians, however, will want to confirm the diagnosis with various laboratory tests. Those commonly ordered are an electroencephalogram (brain wave test) and x-rays of the head. In fairly typical cases, these two tests are all that are necessary. More extensive computerized x-rays, blood tests, dye injections, spinal taps, and other tests may be required in complicated cases.

The following chart will help to distinguish between real and pseudo seizures.

DIFFERENTIAL DIAGNOSIS BETWEEN REAL AND PSEUDO SEIZURES

A. *SYNCOPE* (simple fainting)	*GRAND MAL*
1. Situational (e.g., standing, after voiding, or brushing hair)	1. Not dependant on situation (but may be associated with lack of sleep or food).
2. In adolescence or preadolescence	2. At any age

3. No trismus or incontinence	3. May have trismus or incontinence
4. May have a few jerking movements	4. Jerking movements are prominent
5. EEG usually normal	5. EEG usually paroxysmal
B. *DAYDREAMING*	*PETIT MAL*
1. Lasts minutes	1. Lasts seconds
2. Eyelids don't flutter	2. Eyelids flutter
3. EEG normal	3. EEG definitely abnormal
C. *AGGRESSIVE OR BIZARRE BEHAVIOR*	*PSYCHOMOTOR SEIZURES*
1. No definite beginning or end	1. Clear difference between seizure and nonseizure state
2. Doesn't end in grand mal	2. May conclude with grand mal
3. No aura or vague aura	3. Aura is clear and repetitive
4. Is influenced by environment	4. Is usually independent of environment
5. EEG usually normal	5. EEG usually abnormal, especially in sleep (24-hour trace may be necessary)
D. *PSEUDO OR HYSTERICAL SEIZURES*	*REAL SEIZURES (GRAND MAL)*
1. Influenced by environment	1. Independent of environment
2. Serves a psychological role (e.g., attention getting)	2. Serves no psychological role
3. Patient will not ordinarily hurt self	3. Patient may inadvertently hurt self
4. EEG usually normal even during seizure	4. EEG usually abnormal

Treatment

Emergency On-Site Treatment

The best treatment for grand mal seizures is to let the child be, let the convulsion run its course, and let the child sleep until he or she awakens on his or her own. Unfortunately, it is almost impossible to keep somebody from rubbing the chest, loosening the clothing, or something else equally ineffective. The more stimulation the child receives, the longer the seizure is apt to last, so the less touching the better. As the seizure is about to end, it is a good idea to turn the child on the side so that any secretions or vomitus will run out of the mouth and not back down the throat.

It is an often-stated medical dictum that patients never die during a convulsion. There is a condition, however, called *status epilepticus,* in which the seizure continues for 15 to 30 minutes or longer. Even in these cases the patient does not die, but there is greater danger of brain damage. The dilemma that often arises is, how long is too long? After what length of time should the child be taken to the nearest hospital emergency room or doctor's office? If the child is still convulsing after five minutes, he or she should be taken to the nearest medical facility and given the proper medication to stop the seizure promptly. This usually consists of some intravenous medication such as a barbiturate or Valium. The other types of epilepsy need no emergency treatment except to prevent the child from harming himself or herself.

Medication for Long-Term Control

Epilepsy can be both the easiest and the most difficult of all diseases to treat. It is extremely capricious. Some cases will respond well to a single harmless medication. Other cases require as many as three or four types of medicine, all given several times a day. In these difficult cases, the medicines themselves usually cause some unpleasant side effects and the attending physician must monitor the child frequently.

The medicine must be continued for at least two to five years. Some neurologists have a standing rule that medications must be given for four years after the last convulsion or seizure. If treatment is stopped too soon, the attacks may return with greater severity. For this reason, some feel it is better not to begin treatment after the first attack. Some physicians follow this policy, reasoning that one seizure does not cause ill effects and it may be possible to save the patient four years of drug therapy and emotional trauma. Some children have one typical grand mal seizure and never have another.

All forms of epilepsy are treated by oral medication. The schedule can usually be arranged so the child need not take any pills during school hours. This is by far the best arrangement. If the physician has sound medical reasons for requiring the child to take a dose during school hours, the school authorities should cooperate. However, the psychological effects on the child are so important that the principal or counselor should have a conference with the parent and explore the possibility of giving all doses at home.

Athletic Competition

Children with well-controlled epilepsy can participate in almost all sports. There are two sports that must be considered dangerous for children with epilepsy: gymnastics (rope climbing, parallel bars, swinging rings, trampolines) and swimming, especially under water. Since some children have a history of seizures on hyperventilation, proper preconditioning is essential.

There is more concern and more controversy over participation in football than in any other sport. A seizure on the playing field would be no more harmful than the same seizure anywhere else, but there is a fear that a head injury may aggravate the preexisting epileptic condition and cause more frequent seizures. Actually, there is no good medical evidence to support this fear. However, the general feeling prevails that a child should be in top physical condition, free of all illness, to play this injury-prone sport. A child with epilepsy who is determined, and who is a valuable player besides, will probably find a way to play. If such is the case, it should be only with full knowledge by all concerned of all risks involved. Sometimes a trial period in middle school can be helpful in deciding future plans so that by high school a decision has already been made and agreed upon.

RABIES

Nature of the Condition

Rabies is an infection of the brain (*encephalitis*) caused by a specific virus which can affect many mammals. The most common domestic animals infected are dogs and cats, but horses, cows, and other livestock are susceptible. The largest reservoir is in wild animals and the animals most commonly affected are skunks, foxes, coyotes, bobcats, raccoons, and bats.

Rodents such as squirrels, hamsters, guinea pigs, gerbils, chipmunks, rats, mice, and rabbits are so rarely infected with rabies that health departments often do not even test these animals when people report that they were bitten, and their bites almost never require antirabies treatment.

Exposure and School Relevance

Most commonly, exposure is caused by an animal bite. A nonbite exposure, however, can come from a scratch, abrasion, or other open wound or sore contaminated with animal saliva. Excluding these, a casual contact such as petting a rabid animal is not considered an exposure. (Airborne exposure, as in a bat cave, is very rare; only two cases have been reported.)

Bats are a frequent cause for concern, but it is extremely rare for a bat to bite. There are no vampire bats—the only variety that actually bites—in the United States. Frequently at school, children will pick up a dead bat and play with it. These bats should be sent to the local health department for examination. If rabies virus is found in the bat's brain, each child who played with it must be evaluated individually by a physician to determine the need for rabies vaccine.

Treatment

Management of Biting Animal

Because the disease is so horrible and fatal, any suspected exposure must be handled without compromise. Should a child be bitten on the school grounds by a domestic animal, it is important for the animal to be chained or placed in an escape-proof cage and observed for 10 days. The incubation period of rabies in an animal is less than two weeks. Therefore, if symptoms do not develop in 10 to 14 days, it is safe to assume the animal is not rabid. If a previously healthy dog or cat develops rabies, one of the first things it often does is run away. Therefore, if a child has been bitten by an animal that cannot be found, it must be assumed that the child has been exposed to rabies, and antirabies vaccine must be given.

If a domestic animal develops symptoms of rabies, it should be humanely killed and the head packed in ice until the brain can be examined for rabies. Previously, it was necessary to wait for the animal to die of rabies before examining the brain. Current techniques enable rabies to be identified in the brain at any stage of the disease.

Nothing is more important than identifying the animal and catching it. The police should be notified immediately. Capture and observation of a domestic animal is better than killing it. No matter how small the chance that the animal was sick, no matter how much pity the parent has for the child needing shots, an alternative is not to be considered. The same is true in deciding whether or not to destroy a much-loved pet. Wild animals should be killed and the heads examined as soon as possible.

Management of the Bite

Immediate and thorough washing of the wound using lots of water is very effective and in all probability prevents some cases of rabies, especially in nonbite exposures.

The child should be referred to a physician as soon as possible. Many decisions must be made, such as what type of antirabies vaccine should be used and which child needs treatment. Modern treatment usually consists of 5 or 6 injections, in contrast to the previously required 14 to 21.

Rabies Vaccine

The original rabies vaccine was made from the spinal cord of rabid monkeys. It was effective but the rate of adverse reactions was high. One of the most serious reactions was a permanent paralysis of the legs and occasionally death from paralysis of the respiratory muscles.

Vaccine grown in duck eggs became available in the mid-1950s. It is more effective in preventing rabies and the incidence of serious reaction is much lower.

More recently, a vaccine grown in human cells has become available, and so far it has not only proved the most effective in preventing rabies, but serious reactions have not been reported. It is called human diploid cell vaccine or HDCV.

Rabies immune globulin is also available and is usually used in conjunction with HDCV.

CEREBRAL PALSY

Nature of the Condition

Cerebral palsy is a relatively common disorder seen in schools. It is caused by disease of the brain itself. In most cases, the brain is damaged by disease or injury during fetal life, during the birth process, or shortly after birth.

The nervous system includes the brain, spinal cord, and peripheral nerves. Nerves originate in the brain, go down the spinal cord, and then diverge throughout the body. If a nerve is damaged in the brain or spinal cord, the muscle it supplies becomes fixed in spasm. If that same nerve is damaged after emerging from the spinal cord, the muscle it supplies becomes paralyzed in flaccidity. (Diseases of the peripheral nerves, such as poliomyelitis, produce a flaccid paralysis.)

Since the primary damage is in the brain, the muscles controlled by that part of the brain are paralyzed, but they are fixed in spasm and the child is said to have a spastic paralysis. For this reason, many victims of cerebral palsy are referred to as *spastics*.

Cerebral palsy results from damage to the motor areas, the parts of the brain that send messages out to the muscles—not the part of the brain that receives messages through the sense organs. This concept is basic to an understanding of the difficult life of many of these victims, at least half of whom have good intelligence and an understanding of everything that is going on around them but no way of communicating that understanding.

Symptoms

The nerves that control the muscles of speech, facial expression, and coordinated and controlled arm and leg movement, and those that hold the body in an upright position, all originate in the motor areas of the brain. These nerves are damaged at their very point of origin, and messages transmitted are garbled in severe and bizarre ways. A child who wants to smile may grimace; if the child tries to cry, he or she may smile or laugh or emit weird sounds. Drooling is frequent. The child may be completely unable to speak or be completely unintelligible.

Arm, leg, and trunk muscle involvement causes limping, shuffling gait, unwanted and uncoordinated movements, and falling to the ground.

Generalized convulsions are common, as are convulsions of individual arms and/or legs.

General intelligence or IQ varies considerably; some children are of average or superior intelligence, while others are severely retarded. Testing is often very difficult and frequently requires special skills and special tests.

Classification

1. *Hemiplegia.* Only one side of the body is involved. The arm is usually less useful than the leg, though the child

almost always walks with some limp. This is the most common form.

2. *Monoplegia.* Rarely, only one extremity is involved. In most cases, involvement of the other extremity on the same side can be demonstrated with stress tests.
3. *Quadriplegia.* All four extremities are involved, but usually the legs are worse than the arms.
4. *Paraplegia.* Only the legs are involved.
5. *Diplegia.* All four extremities are involved, with very little noticeable arm involvement.
6. *Athetosis.* This produces unwanted and uncontrollable bizarre body, extremity, and/or facial movements.
7. *Dystonia.* Uncontrollable body muscle tone results in abnormal body postures.
8. *Ataxia.* The child has difficulty or inability to sit or stand upright, or move without holding on.
9. *Atonia.* The child is very limp with no muscle tone. This is very rare and mainly seen in infants.
10. *Mixed.* This form includes various mixtures of the above.

School Relevance

Many children with cerebral palsy can attend regular classes. They will obviously need some help, both academically and physically.

Cerebral palsy can be so severe as to preclude standing, walking, or learning any self-help skills such as feeding or using the toilet. On the other hand, the condition can be so mild that the child is just thought to be excessively clumsy. In these latter cases, the true diagnosis may not be made for many years. Indeed, neurologists sometimes disagree on whether or not a particular child has cerebral palsy.

Treatment

There are five basic forms of treatment:

1. *Medications* are used primarily to control convulsions. All of the various medications used in epilepsy are available. Sometimes, medication will be used to control spasm.

2. *Surgery* is used to lengthen short muscles or tendons and to reinsert tendons into different locations to increase utility of the arms or legs. Many other surgical procedures are beneficial.
3. *Physiotherapy* is useful in almost all cases of cerebral palsy. The earlier it is started, the better the results, and it should be in place long before children start school.
4. *Occupational therapy* helps children learn the skills of daily living, such as sitting, feeding, and writing. This should begin as early as physiotherapy.
5. *Counseling* is necessary for parents as well as children. Both have great need for psychological support and help in a school situation. Counselors who are themselves handicapped often make excellent therapists.

Role of the School Nurse

Obviously, in very mild cases the school nurse will need do no more than for the regular school child. However, most cases will require special nursing knowledge and procedures.

1. *Charting.* Extra care will be required for medication, physiotherapy, and other nursing procedures. The school nurse should keep a chart somewhat similar to a hospital chart that will provide a daily or weekly log.

2. *Medication.* A large proportion of children with cerebral palsy receive medication; many have difficulty swallowing. The school nurse should give the medication and record each dose. The nurse also needs to be aware of adverse reactions to the medicines; a current copy of the PDR (*Physician's Desk Reference*) should be available.

3. *Coordination of physiotherapy and occupational therapy at home and at school.* In many cases therapy is given only at the school or only at the medical office. The school nurse can be instrumental in coordination of services.

4. *Counseling.* In cooperation with the school guidance counselor, the nurse can help the parent accept the child's condition and not continue to seek miracle cures. At the same time, parents must be encouraged to continue therapies that are known to be beneficial.

DEVELOPMENTAL DYSPRAXIA

This is a relatively rare neurological disorder that is also called the *clumsy child syndrome*. All school nurses and teachers will see these children during their careers. The brain pathology is different from that of cerebral palsy, but there is an obvious problem with muscular coordination in this condition also. These children are more than a little clumsy, and they also have a higher than normal incidence of learning problems.

Children who are mentally retarded may also be clumsy. The dyspraxic child is assumed to have normal general intelligence, even though he or she may perform poorly in school. These children will have their greatest problems as they approach ten to twelve years of age, as this is when normal children begin to become quite skillful in athletics. Physical education teachers need to be especially alert to such children because they will need a great deal of encouragement and special tasks commensurate with their ability. Some of the common characteristics of this condition include an awkward and shambling gait, frequent falls when running, poor dressing ability, spilling milk, messy eating, very poor handwriting, slow reaction time, and poor ability in almost any type of organized or competitive sport.

PROGRESSIVE DISEASES OF THE NERVOUS SYSTEM

Nature of the Condition

The word *progressive* indicates an ongoing disease process during which the symptoms get worse. Examples of such diseases are multiple sclerosis, poliomyelitis, brain tumor, and encephalitis. Physicians frequently refer to this group of diseases as progressive central nervous system disease.

Symptoms

The specific symptoms of progressive disease vary greatly. For example, encephalitis or meningitis can cause a child to become severely ill overnight, whereas a brain tumor or multiple sclerosis can progress very slowly. In all cases, however, the disease becomes steadily worse, albeit sometimes very slowly.

School Relevance and Role of the School Nurse

There are certain conditions in which the earliest symptoms that can be seen are subtle changes in the higher cognitive functions such as short-term memory, arithmetic ability, or abstract reasoning. If the motor area of the brain is involved, a change in writing or athletic ability may be noticed.

Since progressive nervous system disease of subtle onset is quite rare, caution should be exercised in notifying parents about such symptoms. However, if a change from previous abilities or a noticeable change in behavior occurs, it would be well for the school nurse to speak with the parent. This may lead to an early diagnosis and thus render the disease a bit more amenable to treatment.

Treatment

Progressive disease is always treated by a physician; the specific treatment is always dependent on the diagnosis.

SECTION 8

SPECIAL SCHOOL-RELATED CONTAGIOUS DISEASES

This section covers the nature, school relevance, symptoms, diagnosis, and treatment of infectious mononucleosis and two different types of hepatitis—chemical or toxic hepatitis and viral hepatitis. It also discusses prevention techniques and the question of giving gamma globulin to school contacts of a child stricken with hepatitis.

In addition, this section briefly discusses the school relevance and transmission of venereal disease, and provides specific information on the nature, symptoms, and treatment of syphilis, gonorrhea, nonspecific urethritis, and others.

INFECTIOUS MONONUCLEOSIS

Nature of the Condition

This relatively common disease, sometimes called glandular fever or mono, is caused by a virus that is related to the herpes simplex virus. Technically, it is called the Epstein–Barr or EB virus. In contrast to the virus of herpes simplex, which causes fever blisters around the mouth and genital area, there is no suspected association with an increased incidence of cancer.

In younger children, the disease is usually mild, probably because the virus is transferred by way of the fingertips and involves small amounts of saliva, whereas young adults get more severe disease from kissing (it is sometimes called the *kissing disease*). The incubation period is usually 30 to 50 days in all age groups. It is seen more commonly in families living in poor socioeconomic circumstances.

School Relevance

Many seem to regard infectious mononucleosis as a more serious disease than it really is. The mortality rate is extremely low, less than in natural measles. The incidence of serious complications (encephalitis and hepatitis) is also quite low. The disease confers a permanent immunity, so second attacks are rare. Apart from its somewhat prolonged course, it is a disease that should occasion no alarm. One often hears of people being tired, rundown, or otherwise chronically incapacitated for months or even years following a bout of infectious mononucleosis. This is a common misconception. Though the disease lasts relatively long, if there are no serious complications, and symptoms of fatigue and lethargy persist longer than one to two months, other causes for that tired feeling should be suspected.

Symptoms and Diagnosis

The most prominent symptoms of the disease are a severe sore throat with marked enlargement of the lymph nodes or glands in the neck, and lesser enlargement of the glands in the rest of the body. There is always a fever, usually high, and sometimes a measles-like rash.

Infectious mononucleosis lasts longer than most contagious diseases in children; often, the fever will last 10 to 14 days and a feeling of weakness and tiredness may persist for several weeks. For this reason, and because the disease may be quite mild in younger children, an incorrect diagnosis is often made in children who have a mild sore throat with low-grade fever that lasts more than 6 or 7 days. Several reliable laboratory tests are available; there is now a direct test for the virus itself, so errors in diagnosis should be much less common.

Treatment

There is no specific antibiotic that has a curative effect, though antibiotics are often prescribed because of severe tonsillitis. Bed rest and a high fluid intake are helpful. Younger children who feel well may be allowed the freedom of the house but should not play outdoors.

HEPATITIS

Nature of the Condition

Hepatitis simply means disease of the liver. It can be caused by chemicals, viruses, bacteria, fungi, or other agents.

All types of hepatitis share various symptoms to some degree. In some types, certain symptoms are more severe than others; for example, a large, painful, tender liver with no jaundice in some infections and extreme jaundice with little or no tenderness or pain in others.

Types

Chemical or Toxic Hepatitis

Among the many toxic substances that damage the liver—DDT, chloroform, carbon tetrachloride, and so on—the most widespread by far is alcohol. Alcohol is metabolized in the liver, but in excess it acts as a poison and damages the liver cells. Many chronic alcoholics eventually get toxic hepatitis after many years of drinking.

Viral Hepatitis

Although viral hepatitis has a low incidence—in a school of 500 students, one will perhaps see about five cases a year—it causes great anxiety, because almost everyone has heard about a rare fatal case. While there is no specific treatment, many supportive measures are available, and with proper care fatalities are very rare. Also, an understanding of how it is transmitted should somewhat allay the fears that teachers and parents so often express. Actually, because of its nature of transmission, it is rarely caught at school. There are at least three different types of viral hepatitis:

1. Infectious hepatitis, or hepatitis A
2. Serum hepatitis, or hepatitis B
3. A recently discovered type that is neither of the above, which has not yet been named—currently called non-A, non-B viral hepatitis.

1. *Hepatitis A.* This is caused by oral ingestion of a specific virus, and transmission is by the fecal–oral route. Any mechanism that can cause human sewage or fecal material of any sort to enter the water or food supply can be a source of infection. People with virus in their stools can transmit it by way of their fingers (failure to wash hands after a bowel movement). Evidence has accumulated that indicates that a reservoir of viral hepatitis A exists in

day-care centers catering to children under the age of two years (obviously related to diaper changing). The incubation period (the time between ingestion of the virus and the earliest onset of symptoms) is 15 to 45 days. **Almost all cases in school children are of this type.**

The most contagious stage is in the late incubation period, so that by the time jaundice develops and the diagnosis is made, the disease is rapidly becoming less contagious even though the patient may be getting sicker.

2. *Hepatitis B.* This was previously thought to occur only following blood transfusions; now much more is known about it. It is caused by a completely different virus from that of hepatitis A. In infected individuals, hepatitis B virus can be found in urine, saliva, semen, bile, vaginal secretions, blood, and some other body fluids. It is rarely present in feces.

The best-known method of transmission is transfusion with infected blood or accidentally pricking a finger (if one is a lab technician). However, it is now known that sexual activity can also transmit the disease. Prostitutes have a very high level of antibodies against this disease, indicating past infection.

Hepatitis B, in contrast to A, has a much longer incubation period—one to six months—and chronic carriers are much more common; thus, it is thought that there is a pool of about one million active carriers in the United States. The symptoms themselves are similar to those of hepatitis A, and it can require sophisticated laboratory work and good clinical detection to be able to tell one from the other.

3. *Non-A, Non-B Hepatitis.* Most post-transfusion hepatitis is of this variety. It can cause a chronic carrier state and can also be acquired through sexual activity, much like hepatitis B.

Symptoms and Diagnosis

1. Early—fever, malaise (feeling sick), loss of appetite, and stomach ache.
2. One to two days later—continuation of early symptoms plus nausea and vomiting.

3. About same time or one or two days later—jaundice plus continuation of other symptoms.

The severity of illness is usually age related—children often have milder disease. Therefore, many children develop *anicteric hepatitis (icterus* is a medical word for jaundice), which means that they have the disease but no jaundice. The whites of the eyes offer the easiest and earliest place to detect yellow discoloration. A child with very mild disease may have only a three- to five-day illness with low fever, loss of appetite, nausea, and a little stomach ache. Then the child gets well. Many of these children don't even stay home from school, and nobody ever knows they had hepatitis. They are, of course, just as contagious. Half of the population over the age of 50 has antibodies against hepatitis A, meaning that they had the disease at some earlier time in their lives. One attack usually confers lifetime immunity, and there are no chronic carriers. Rarely is the disease severe, and the overall mortality rate is less than 1 percent.

School Relevance

Many teachers and school administrators view hepatitis with more fear than it deserves. It is true that there are fatal cases, but they are extremely rare; there are more fatalities from measles. Many teachers are immune to hepatitis because of minimal contact with the virus in childhood.

Some schools institute a massive cleaning program each time a case of hepatitis is discovered in the school. While it makes sense to wash doorknobs, handles, and other objects that are customarily touched with the hands, it doesn't help to scrub floors or spray walls or rooms. This is expensive, and some sprays are actually dangerous.

In most states, hepatitis is a reportable disease; confirmed cases should be reported to the local public health authorities. Some school districts send notice to parents when a case of hepatitis occurs. This allows parents to seek advice from a doctor or the school nurse when they learn that their child may have been exposed. (See sample letter on page 279.)

Prevention

Handwashing

If everyone always washed their hands after a bowel movement and if no one ever put their hands to their faces, there would be very little hepatitis in children. This is by far the most effective way to prevent the spread of hepatitis A. Unfortunately, in spite of all exhortations, this has not occurred and there is no reason to suspect that we can rely on education alone as the prime method of prevention.

Gamma Globulin (GG)

Hepatitis can be prevented about 90 percent of the time if a dose of 0.02 cc of GG per kilogram of body weight is given intramuscularly within two weeks of exposure. This means that a 150-pound individual would require a dose of about 1½ cc. In some cases, larger doses are used because the doctor may suspect hepatitis B, which requires a dose three times larger or because exposure occurred more than two weeks before the shot is to be given.

There is now available a new and effective vaccine that prevents hepatitis B. It is very expensive and is recommended only for certain high-risk individuals. A physician should make the decision.

The question of whether to give school contacts a shot of GG always arises. The answer is usually no if the exposure is only in the classroom. For special close friends who play together every day, or for siblings, the doctor usually suggests that it be given. There are two things to remember. One is that each case is individual, and the child's personal physician should make the decision. There are dozens of extenuating circumstances that go into the final decision of whether or not to administer GG and how much to give. Second, most school-contact children do not need it. Here is what the American Academy of Pediatrics has to say about hepatitis A:

> It is a disease that is not very contagious (compared to measles, etc.) and therefore, it is unusual for two cases to

occur in the same classroom. It is usually mild in children. It is caused by a virus that may be found in secretions of the mouth and nose, but is especially found in the urine and stool of the person with the disease. Therefore, washing the hands after going to the bathroom is especially important. Protection with gamma globulin is recommended only for certain household contacts and people living in institutions such as orphanages, asylums, etc.

Treatment

There is no specific treatment for viral hepatitis; there is no antibiotic or antiviral medicine that actually kills the virus. Therefore, preventive measures are of paramount importance. There are many supportive measures that are helpful, however:

1. *Rest.* In the early stages it is important for children to be in bed or at least indoors, depending on the severity of the disease.
2. *Food.* Since loss of appetite and nausea are prominent symptoms, it is difficult for the child to eat the foods necessary to fortify the liver. Small amounts of appetizing carbohydrates at frequent intervals are helpful.
3. *Fluids.* All types of liquids are helpful, and in the early stages of the illness the child may not tolerate much else without vomiting.

VENEREAL DISEASE

School Relevance

Modern society talks about and engages in sexual practices much more than in the past. Promiscuity has affected the student population as well. More individuals are sexually active at a younger age and with a greater variety of partners. This has caused venereal disease (VD) to leap to epidemic numbers. Whereas in the past VD meant syphilis and gonorrhea, the rapidly rising number of cases has caused previously rare conditions to be added to the list of sexually transmitted diseases. Herpes simplex, hepatitis B, and several lesser-known diseases are seen more and more commonly.

In spite of the serious threat this presents to school children, there is still widespread opposition to presenting effective education in the schools to offer the students information that could protect them from such exposure. The assumption is that if the students hear about sex, they will get ideas. In actual fact, they have already heard about it. Lots of them are past the idea stage. Those students who are not sexually active have made the choice for abstinence in spite of the fact that they have heard about sex. How simple it would be if society could view VD as dispassionately as it now does tuberculosis! Then methods of reporting and treating existing cases would become more effective, causing the incidence to drop.

Unfortunately, most current attempts at sex education resemble the scare tactics used in the late 1960s and early 1970s, which tried to dissuade young people from using marijuana. A common approach to sex education is to invite a guest speaker from some agency to show a film during gym to some 40 to 60 students of the same sex. The movie preaches sexual abstinence, depicts the horrors of various venereal diseases, and describes the treatment for these illnesses. This is followed by a question-and-answer period. Unfortunately, this message has not had the desired effect in junior and senior high schools, where the incidence of venereal disease increases annually. It is doubtful that current health education methods will work. To be effective, this type of education would have to embrace the wider area of sexuality in general, consider the negative aspects of recreational sex, emphasize emotional love and responsibility over hormonal urges, and, above all, it would have to be built on some simple, basic knowledge of anatomy and physiology. This will not happen until society urges schools to incorporate this kind of teaching, beginning in the late elementary grades, and until colleges begin training teachers who can teach it. Such effective sex education will help control not only venereal disease but many other problems connected with contemporary sexual practices.

Routes of Transmission

In spite of the fact that it is theoretically possible for any venereal disease to be transmitted by nonvenereal means, in actual practice it is very rare for an individual to contact any venereal disease other than by some form of direct sexual activity—in particular, direct mouth-to-mouth kissing or direct genital contact, either heterosexual or homosexual. Contracting venereal disease from a toilet seat or drinking glass or any other intermediate object is largely a myth; it is theoretically possible and undoubtedly some cases exist, but very few have been documented outside of the laboratory worker who accidentally pricks his or her finger with a needle containing infected blood or serum.

SYPHILIS

Nature of the Condition

Syphilis has plagued humankind since antiquity. It has existed for so many centuries that it seems the human race has developed a partial immunity to it. Several hundred years ago, *spirocheta pallida,* the germ that causes syphilis, was so virulent that it occasionally caused a high fever, delirium, coma, and death within a week.

Symptoms and Stages

Primary

The primary lesion usually consists of a genital sore (*chancre*) that goes away untreated in one to three weeks. There may or may not be a low-grade fever, but the affected individual is not very sick. Since the chancre is relatively painless, the doctor is often not even consulted though the disease is highly contagious. The chancre is usually located on the glans penis (the tip end), the labia minora (the inner vaginal lips), and rarely on the tonsil or adjacent to the rectal opening.

Secondary

The secondary stage of syphilis occurs about six to eight weeks later and can manifest itself in various forms. A common finding is a nonitching skin rash that looks like mild measles. Whitish patches sometimes occur inside the mouth and are called *mucus patches.* They are highly contagious, especially through kissing. This stage is usually accompanied by fever and malaise. It usually goes away untreated in one to three weeks. There are many other possible manifestations of secondary syphilis, such as acute meningitis or encephalitis, different kinds of skin rashes, bald spots, and arthritis. Occasionally, secondary symptoms continue to reappear for six to nine months or for as long as two years.

Tertiary

The first two stages are almost always benign and self-limiting. The third or tertiary stage occurs five to twenty years later. It has become quite rare since the availability of penicillin. The tertiary stage in untreated syphilis occurs in only about 25 to 30 percent of individuals who have had the primary or secondary stage. It can attack the brain, spinal cord, heart, or other organs. In any case, the illness and damage caused by the tertiary stage are usually very serious and sometimes fatal.

Treatment

The treatment today is extremely simple and effective. The first effective treatment was a form of arsenic developed by Paul Ehrlich. It was called salvarsan, was quite toxic, required a two- to three-year course of treatment, and did not work too well. Treatment methods were gradually refined and arsenic preparations improved, so that by about 1940 one could cure many cases of early syphilis (primary or secondary) with a six-month course of quite painful injections of a new type of arsenic and bismuth. Nowadays, most early syphilis can be cured dependably with a single shot of the proper dose of penicillin. This represents one of the most dramatic miracle cures ever wrought by medical science.

GONORRHEA

Nature of the Condition

Gonorrhea, now one of the most common communicable diseases in the world except for the common cold, is also one of the classical venereal diseases of antiquity. It is commonly called *the clap* and is caused by a germ called *Neisseria gonorrhea* or simply the gonococcus. It settles in the urethra in males and in the cervix in females, producing a purulent (pus) discharge plus various other symptoms. The time between exposure and first onset of symptoms can be two to ten days, but in most cases it is about two to four days.

Symptoms

In males this infection causes burning on urination. In females the infection is often painless, but if it spreads up into the uterus and fallopian tubes, it can cause intense abdominal pain. Further serious complications such as peritonitis may ensue if treatment is delayed. Also, complications can occur in males, especially if the infection travels to the testicles or prostate gland.

In recent years the gonococcus has been found in the throat and rectum in increasing numbers of patients who regularly indulge in oral or anal sex practices, either homosexual or heterosexual.

In both males and females, either because of partial natural immunity or partial treatment, the urethral or vaginal discharge can diminish to such a small amount that it is almost unnoticeable and completely painless. It is, however, just as contagious. Gonorrhea has become unchallenged as the most prevalent of all serious venereal diseases, and the incidence is rising each year.

Treatment

Treatment is quite simple; a single injection of penicillin will cure most early cases, but most physicians prescribe a combination of medications. The gonococcus tends to develop a resistance against antibiotic action, and there are many strains of the germ that are partially or completely penicillin-resistant. If complications ensue, a longer course of treatment is usually required along with bed rest.

NONSPECIFIC URETHRITIS AND OTHER GENITAL INFECTIONS

Nature of the Condition

In addition to the gonococcus, there are many germs, viruses, and fungi that can cause infections in the urethra, vagina, cervix, or other genital organs. Taken as a group, infections with any of these agents have been labeled nonspecific urethritis or nonspecific genital disease. In some cases, the causative organism can be identified.

At the present time, the known causative agents of genitourinary disease, all of which are capable of being spread by sexual contact, are:

1. *Trichomonas*—a one-celled animal organism (related to the amoeba)
2. *Monilia*—a yeast-like fungus
3. *Chlamydia*—a combination virus–bacterium
4. *Herpes simplex*—a pure virus

The first three of the above cause only a mild vaginal or urethral discharge. The fourth—herpes virus—causes sores that burn or itch. This is the same virus that causes fever blisters around the nose and lips and can also cause similar sores on the penis (usually the tip end) or around the cervix. These sores itch and burn and are readily spread by sexual contact. In addition to the burning and itching, it is suspected that women with herpes infections of the cervix are more prone to develop cancer of the cervix.

Symptoms

Generally speaking, these diseases usually cause a mild urethral or vaginal discharge, some itching, plus a small amount of burning on urination. In almost all cases, the degree of symptoms is less than in gonorrhea. Also, complications rarely occur. Since a small amount of vaginal discharge is normal, a woman with a very mild nonspecific vaginitis may be unaware of her infection yet fully capable of passing it on to her sexual partner. Also, the male can unknowingly harbor certain organisms in his urethra without developing any noticeable symptoms but be capable of infecting his sexual partner. A married couple may continue to give the infection to each other unless both are treated simultaneously, even though only one (usually the female) may manifest symptoms.

There are two types of herpes virus. Type I is found about the nose and lips, and type II is in the genital area. They can be differentiated with certain laboratory tests, and it is now known that type I virus can also infect the genital area with oral–genital contact. (See Section 2.)

With good methods of detection, the cause can be identified in about 60 to 70 percent of all cases of mild genitourinary infection. That leaves 30 to 40 percent of nonspecific disease for which no cause can be found.

Treatment

Treatment varies depending on the causative organism. Chlamydia, trichomonas, and monilia can all be treated quite effectively. There is as yet no effective cure for herpes infection though many agents have been tried. The remaining venereal disease, those that are truly nonspecific (cause unknown), are treated by cleanliness, time, and educated guesses.

OTHER VENEREAL DISEASES

Nature of the Condition

Diseases spread by venereal contact, in the United States as in other parts of the world, exist in larger numbers than many people are aware. The less common are unknown to most people and the average doctor rarely sees them. They are commonly seen in VD clinics.

Generally speaking, they cause various kinds of surface lesions (sores, warts, lymph node swellings, etc.) in the genital area, and occasionally more serious complications ensue. These diseases are:

1. *Lymphogranuloma venereum*
2. *Chancroid* (soft chancre)
3. *Condyloma acuminata* (venereal warts)
4. *Granuloma inguinale*
5. *Reiter's disease*
6. *Hepatitis B*
7. *AIDS* (acquired immune deficiency syndrome)

Hepatitis is now considered a venereal disease because the virus is present in semen, saliva, and vaginal secretion, so it is theoretically possible to contact it through kissing or heterosexual intercourse. In actual practice, however, almost all cases of sexually acquired hepatitis B have been the result of anal intercourse; therefore, most cases occur in male homosexuals. This is probably caused by some tearing and bleeding of the rectal lining so that there is direct bloodstream contamination. (See "Hepatitis" in this section.)

AIDS, though uncommon, has assumed great notoriety in recent years because of its high mortality rate. It is presumed to be caused by a virus, though none has yet been identified. It is spread in much the same manner as hepatitis B and found in the same groups of individuals—male homosexuals, lab workers, and those receiving frequent blood transfusions. It will rarely be seen in a school child. Because the route of transmission is similar to that of hepatitis B, school personnel need have no fear of contracting it during school hours.

Some of these less common venereal diseases are readily treatable, and some are not. In all cases, a specialist in venereal diseases needs to be consulted.

Concerns of the Teacher and the Principal

Obviously, it is never necessary to exclude a pupil from school because of VD, even in the unlikely event that its existence should become known. None of the other students or faculty is in any danger of contracting the disease in a nonvenereal way.

Frequently, the local health department, in its case-finding efforts, will contact a school official to report that one of the students in that school has been named as a contact. This often happens when another student, following the appearance of certain alarming symptoms, goes directly to the health department for diagnosis and treatment, not only bypassing the family physician, but the family as well. The law now permits the health department to treat these youngsters without parental consent. In the course of treatment the infected youngster is asked to name all of the sexual contacts involved so that they can be warned or treated, as the case may be. The health department, to keep the youngster's confidence and preserve his or her privacy, often tries to talk to the named contact at school rather than at home. (Also, it's easier to find children at school.) Often the principal is troubled by someone from outside the school talking to a student about such matters without the parents being aware of what's happening. Naturally, it's better for all concerned if the student is able to tell the parents what has happened and have them cooperate in the treatment. However, as every principal knows, there are many homes in which this type of communication simply cannot and does not take place. In such circumstances, it is far better to have the youngster adequately treated because of the potential dangers of ravaging complications. The principal should arrange a private room where the venereal disease control agent from the health department can talk to the student personally, or arrange a quiet, private, and confidential telephone conversation and then use his or her influence or that of the counselor or school nurse to urge the student to obtain the necessary tests for diagnosis and treatment.

SECTION 9

BITES AND STINGS

This section covers the nature, symptoms, treatment, and school relevance of various kinds of insect stings and bites, and human bites. It also provides suggested guidelines for emergency medication for individuals who have an extreme hypersensitivity to insect stings and recommendations to accompany the insect allergy emergency kit that such individuals often carry.

BEES AND WASPS

Nature of the Condition

The most common insect stings are those of bees and wasps (hornets and mud daubers are varieties of wasps). These stings usually cause a severe pain that diminishes over five to ten minutes, and in fifteen minutes the symptoms have all but gone. While the amount of pain and swelling varies with each individual sting, the types of reactions fall into two major categories.

Symptoms

Local reactions

This type of reaction indicates that the body's immune mechanism is effectively defending against the insect venom and thereby preventing the entire body from reacting adversely. Following are some examples:

1. A small, red, painful, swollen area that becomes normal in ten to fifteen minutes
2. A sting on the hand or foot, causing equal duration of pain, but with the entire hand or foot remaining swollen for several days
3. A sting on the forehead that causes both eyes to swell

Generalized reactions

These occur in a part of the body far removed from the bite. Examples are swelling of the lips and/or eyelids from a bite on the hand, a rash all over the body from a single sting anywhere, or swelling of the hands from a bite on the leg. Reactions of this nature can be dangerous because they indicate that the body has a weak immune mechanism against insect venom and signal the possibility of an increasingly severe reaction to subsequent stings. In the United States, there are about 50 to 60 deaths a year from bee or wasp stings; they are almost all caused by one of the following severe types of generalized reactions:

1. Swelling of the larynx (voice box), the narrowest part of the airway. A small degree of swelling can cause obstruction to respiration.
2. Anaphylactic shock resulting when all of the small blood vessels in the body dilate and cause the blood pressure to drop very quickly. The patient suddenly feels faint, begins to perspire, feels cold, and in a very short time may lose consciousness.

Treatment and School Relevance

The school principal and school nurse should see that the playground and buildings are periodically inspected, and the students should be instructed to report any beehives or wasp nests. Local reactions are best treated with an ice cube or an anesthetic ointment like benzocaine. Another useful household remedy is meat tenderizer that contains an enzyme derived from papaya. (This is also useful to relieve jellyfish or Portuguese man-o'-war stings.) Juice of the aloe vera plant has also been recommended.

If the stinger is present, it should be removed with the fingernail or a knife blade. Since it usually has a tiny venom sac attached, care must be taken not to squeeze it.

In cases of persistent swelling of the hands or feet because of local reactions, it is best to consult a doctor. Though medicine taken internally is rarely necessary for local reactions, on occasion it may be required.

Since generalized reactions are always potentially serious, it is advisable to consult a physician. Most allergists recommend a series of desensitization shots and in addition request that the patient carry a small kit containing adrenalin, an antihistamine, and a needle and syringe. (See Figure 9–1.) With proper prevention and treatment, almost all severe or fatal reactions can be avoided.

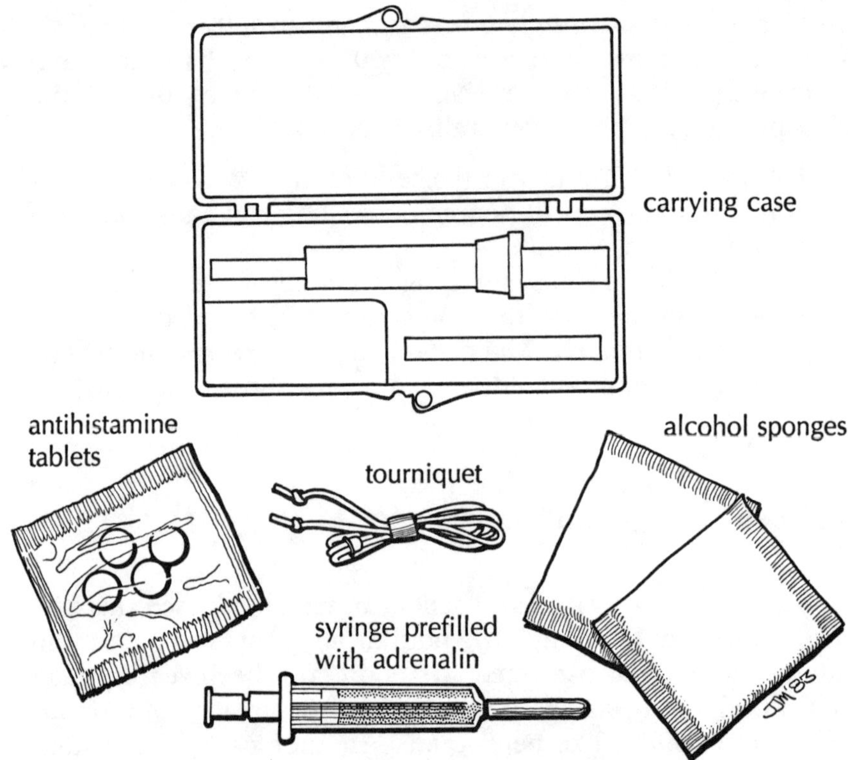

Figure 9–1. Emergency insect sting kit

The school principal should allow this kit to be kept in a refrigerator and should make it readily accessible to the child, the school nurse, or whoever is designated to give the injection when necessary. In cases of this nature it is well to establish contact with the child's physician. A sample form follows.

GUIDELINES FOR EMERGENCY SCHOOL TREATMENT

Emergency Medication—Injectable and/or Oral
For Extreme and Dangerous Hypersensitivity to Insect Sting

Extreme hypersensitivity to insect sting is a potentially life-threatening situation. Many physicians ask these patients to carry an emergency kit containing injectable adrenalin (epinephrin) and/or an oral medicine.

Since this problem is rare but potentially extremely dangerous, we urge school district superintendents, school nurses, and physicians to be aware of the problem and, to as full an extent as possible, follow the proposed suggestions.

I. Suggestions to the school district

1. The school district should accept an emergency insect sting kit prescribed by a physician if certain conditions are met as outlined below. The emergency kit should be kept where the child and a responsible adult can reach it fast.
2. The school district should allow the school nurse, if the nurse is on campus, to give an emergency injection at school in cases when the physician has met certain criteria outlined below.
3. The school district should allow the child to give himself or herself the injection if it has been properly prescribed and the physician has met the criteria outlined below.
4. Other campus personnel, previously identified as capable of giving shots, may be allowed to give the emergency injection if the school nurse is absent and the child cannot give it to himself or herself.
5. If the school nurse is not present, the child cannot give himself or herself the medication, and nobody is available to give it, the child should be evacuated by EMS or other more feasible method as soon as he or she reports having been stung.

II. Suggestions for the school nurse

1. The nurse should give the injectable and/or oral medicine, as ordered, as soon as the child reports he or she has been stung. The nurse should not wait to observe any reactions.
2. The school nurse should recommend that the child be evacuated as soon as possible after the first dose of oral and/or injectable medicine.
3. If the child has not yet been evacuated, in 15 minutes the school nurse may give a second dose of oral and/or injectable medication provided it has been so prescribed by the physician.

III. Suggestions for the physician

1. The school nurse will follow your orders as closely as the state Nurse Practice Act permits.

2. The school nurse can give emergency medication—oral and/or injectable—if school district policy permits.
3. The school nurse *cannot* observe a child for symptoms and then make a decision about whether to give or withhold oral or injectable medication. The nurse must give the medication immediately upon report of the sting and at such times (10 to 15 minutes) immediately after as prescribed.
4. It is strongly recommended that the physician notify the school principal by telephone in each case, explain the situation, and ask to have the school nurse call back.
5. The physician must send short, clear written instructions with each emergency kit in addition to the above phone call.

SAMPLE RECOMMENDATIONS TO ACCOMPANY INSECT ALLERGY EMERGENCY KIT

_______(name)_______is highly allergic to the stings of bees, wasps, and ants and needs the following emergency care when stung:

1. Chew two tablets of chlortrimeton.
2. Give shot:______cc of adrenalin.
3. Remove stinger if obvious. Remove the stinger from the wound if it is still present. Use fine tweezers, long fingernails, or a knife blade to scrape off the stinger. Do not grasp any fleshy portion of the venom sack, for it will inject more venom.
4. Use ice pads. Apply an ice pack, if available, to slow the absorption.
5. Go to emergency room or doctor's office.
6. Give second shot—same dose—in 15 minutes if still at school.

Please review these instructions every two or three months and check the epinephrin (adrenalin) at that time. Check expiration date. It must be replaced if any color develops or particles appear in the fluid. Refrigeration is not necessary, but avoid prolonged exposure to heat, such as in a closed car or in direct sun.

Do not discard the syringe or medicine vials, but take them with you to the emergency room or doctor's office in order that they can be sure of exactly what you've done.

Please call our office and report results of stings at your convenience.

FIRE ANTS AND OTHER INSECTS

This type of mound-building ant is found mostly in the southern states. While the bite is quite painful, it rarely causes the serious generalized type of reaction described above. This ant's chief danger is to small children who may inadvertently stand in an ant bed and receive so many bites that the total envenomation is serious. Rare fatalities have been reported in children and animals.

Many caterpillars, notably the Italian asp, cause a type of sting from venom on their feet. Earwigs, scorpions, and other miscellaneous insects can bite or sting.

Treatment is always the same as for local reactions to bee stings. In cases of multiple fire ant bites, especially in a small child, immediate consultation with a physician is advisable.

SPIDERS

Spiders (not technically insects) rarely bite humans. There are only two that are of any concern: the brown recluse and the black widow. Both types of bites need to be treated by a physician and should be referred as promptly as possible. Ice should be applied at school.

HUMAN BITES

Because of the large number of bacteria that live in the mouth, human bites—more than any other variety—are likely to become infected.

Therefore, careful and prolonged washing, preferably with an antibacterial soap (betadine, for example), is necessary. Following thorough cleansing, a loose dressing should be applied so that air can reach the abraded surface.

If the bite is minimal, daily washing will suffice to cure it. If it is worse, it should be referred to a physician.

SECTION 10

DIABETES

The special problems of diabetic students are discussed in this section. Included are a description of diabetes and steps for its diagnosis and effective treatment.

Nature of the Condition

Diabetes mellitus, or sugar diabetes, is a disease of one part of the pancreas (sweetbreads in cattle), a gland located near the stomach. This part of the gland secretes two hormones: insulin and glucagon. These two hormones regulate the blood's sugar level; insulin causes the blood sugar level to go down, and glucagon causes it to go up.

Patients with diabetes do not produce enough insulin; therefore, their blood sugar level goes up. As the blood sugar level rises, other changes occur that, in childhood, cause rapidly progressive severe symptoms.

There are two types of diabetes: type I or juvenile-onset diabetes, and type II or adult-onset diabetes. On occasion an older person (over 35) will develop type I diabetes, and very rarely a child will develop type II diabetes. Type I may be seen at any age in childhood. The peak age of onset is 11 to 13 years. The younger the child, the faster the disease progresses. It is rare in children under three years old.

Symptoms

Type I

The classical symptoms are excessive thirst, urination, appetite, and weight loss. The symptoms can progress quite rapidly, so that in two to four weeks the child becomes thin and dehydrated, progressively weaker, and less responsive, with deep, rapid respirations and, if untreated, coma and death. Associated symptoms are blurred vision, bed wetting, itching, and skin infections.

In addition to the abnormal carbohydrate metabolism, other changes occur in the large and small arteries and the peripheral nerves. These changes, however, take many years to develop and are rarely seen in school children.

Children who develop diabetes are rarely overweight; diet or excessive sugar intake is not the cause. It is inherited as a genetic predisposition.

Type II

This almost always occurs in middle or later life, is associated with diet and obesity, and progresses slowly. It is extremely rare in school-age children, so it will not be dealt with in this section.

Diagnosis

Diabetes is a rare disease, occurring in about one in 2,500 children under age 15. A classical case of childhood diabetes can almost be diagnosed by symptoms alone. The school nurse should be on the lookout for any child who loses weight, especially if he or she continues to eat well. Diabetic children always lose weight; they never simply fail to gain. Many preadolescent children gain weight very slowly—two to four pounds a year—so diabetes need not be suspected if a child simply fails to gain. Blood and urine sugar tests are always performed to confirm the diagnosis and to determine the severity of the disease. Many school nurses now have urine test paper strips, which can be used in suspicious cases.

Special Problems at Adolescence and Emotional Problems

As with any handicapped child, the rebellious adolescent diabetic also presents special problems. It is important for the school nurse to help the child during special situations in school. Teachers may need explanations for rest-room excuses for urine testing. Coaches need to know about the importance of regular amounts of exercise with little change from day to day (the more exercise, the less insulin required—within limits). The principal needs to make allowances for absences; by communication with the physician, the school nurse can help determine which absences are necessary.

Diabetic children who develop hypoglycemia (excessively low blood sugar) are likely to exhibit aggressiveness, irritability, or other behavioral symptoms as their first symptoms. **Any unusual**

behavior in a child with diabetes should arouse suspicions that the child may have an imbalance of blood sugar.

Treatment

Juvenile diabetics (type I) always need insulin; their condition cannot be controlled by diet alone. Oral antidiabetic medications, so commonly used in type II diabetes, should not be used.

The so-called treatment triad consists of:

1. Insulin
2. Diet
3. Exercise

The amount of insulin required varies for each child but always depends on the caloric intake and the amount of exercise. The more food eaten, the more insulin required; the more exercise, the less insulin required.

Insulin. Most children with diabetes will receive two doses a day, both at home; one in the morning and the second between 4:00 and 5:00 P.M. The individual total daily dose will vary from 5 units to 75 or 90 units, depending on many factors. The doctor will determine each child's dose. The school nurse should be alert to events that may require a change in or elimination of a dose. *Warning:* It is always safer to give too little insulin than too much. Too little insulin results in a slow rise in blood sugar with relatively slow onset of serious symptoms. Too much insulin results in a rapid decline in blood sugar with relatively rapid onset of serious symptoms. Whether or not the school nurse is scheduled to give a child a prescribed dose of insulin each day (a rare situation), the nurse must always be able to contact the doctor or doctor's assistant if a situation arises that requires a change in the daily dose.

Diet. The childhood diabetic needs a carefully prescribed diet. It is most important not to become obese. The caloric content should remain steady and only vary within prescribed limits, and the diet should be one that the child enjoys and eats willingly. Special health foods and so-called diabetic foods are never necessary. Missing a meal is not a reason for omitting an insulin dose. It is a reason for finding out why the meal was missed and consultation with the doctor's office. It is not good practice for the child to regularly eat too much and take more insulin to control the resultant rise in blood sugar. It makes the diabetes much more difficult to control. At the same time, it is not emotionally healthy to forbid the after-football-game chocolate ice cream sundae that "all the other kids are having." This type of exception can be, and usually is, easily worked out in advance.

Exercise. In 1935, Dr. E. P. Joslin wrote:

> Exercise tends to lower the blood sugar in the diabetic.... the effect is so striking and so beneficial that exercise ... is now accorded a prominent place in treatment.... Through muscular activity food tolerance improves and higher diets with smaller doses of insulin are possible. This is most strikingly shown in the much lower insulin requirement of diabetic children in summer camp as compared to the larger need when they are in school and relatively inactive.

These words are still true. While regular exercise is important, the preteen child's normal play activities are usually sufficient. It is not necessary to enroll in special exercise, karate, or soccer classes for the sake of the diabetes alone. On the other hand, a sedentary child needs to be encouraged to run, climb, and jump in normal play. Teenage children more often need organized physical activities. In all cases, common sense—with due regard for the child's physical and emotional health—should prevail. It is impossible to control obesity with exercise alone; proper diet is always necessary.

Complications

Hypoglycemia (low blood sugar) is by far the most frequent complication. It is caused by excess insulin in relation to diet and exercise. It comes on rapidly and needs to be managed early before the child loses consciousness.

The early warning signs are sweating, pallor, trembling, rapid pulse, and blurred vision. Later signs are confusion, disorientation, aggressiveness, and partial or complete unconsciousness. As in adults who are are mistaken to be drunk, students may appear drugged. This is also called insulin reaction.

Preferred early treatment is a glass of milk or orange juice. Each contains just enough rapidly absorbable sugar to cause a proper and safe rise in blood sugar. If there is no observable response in five minutes, the child should chew a package of mints, which contains more sugar. If symptoms are not relieved in five to ten minutes, the student must be rushed to the nearest emergency medical facility.

An ideal situation is to have a blood sugar testing kit on each campus. (See below.) A blood sugar reading of less than 60 will show that the student is having an insulin reaction instead of early diabetic acidosis.

Glucagon is commercially available and is excellent for the treatment of insulin reactions. It is given intramuscularly. The usual dose is 1 milligram and is generally considered safe. However, it is sometimes very difficult to differentiate an insulin reaction from early diabetic coma, an opposite type of reaction, in which glucagon should not be given.

On occasion, a doctor will give a patient a prescription for glucagon, instruct the parent to buy it, take it to school, and tell the school nurse to give 1 milligram if the child has an insulin reaction. This is totally unwarranted. A school nurse should not give glucagon unless a physician consultant is readily available, there are signed standing orders, and the nurse has demonstrated proficiency in differentiating insulin reaction from diabetic acidosis (early diabetic coma). Even with all of the foregoing criteria, most school nurses should only give a single dose upon direct telephone order from the physician.

Diabetic acidosis refers to a condition that ensues when the blood sugar rises (because of excessive food intake, too little exercise, or not enough insulin) and the child's diabetes begins to go out of control. The early observable symptoms are somewhat similar to those of an insulin reaction; the child is somewhat confused, disoriented, and semiconscious.

There are differentiating features, however, as shown in the table on page 138.

Urticaria (hives) at the site of insulin injection is fairly common and usually goes away after the first week or two of therapy.

	Hypoglycemia	Diabetic Acidosis
History	Insufficient food, excess insulin, excess exercise	Lack of insulin, stress, GI upset, febrile illness
Onset	Relatively rapid, one to three hours	Relatively slow, four to ten hours or more
Symptoms	Anxiety, sweating, hunger, headache, blurred vision, twitching	Increased thirst and urination, loss of appetite, nausea, vomiting
Physical Findings	Pale moist skin, full rapid pulse, dilated pupils, rising blood pressure	Red dry skin, soft eyeballs, deep rapid breathing, falling blood pressure
Laboratory Findings	Low blood sugar, sugar-free urine	High blood sugar, high urine sugar

Adapted from Textbook of Endocrinology, *Williams, R.H. W.B. Saunders Co., Philadelphia, 1981*

Lipodystrophy or breakdown of fatty tissue at the injection site occurs very often. The long-term prognosis for complete disappearance of these lumpy, soft skin swellings or depressions is excellent, though sometimes they last two to ten years.

Long-term complications consist of artery and nerve tract changes, which may produce symptoms in the eyes, heart, brain, kidneys, and legs. These changes take 12 to 15 years or longer to develop and are rarely seen in school-age children.

The school nurse should be aware that most authorities now agree that patients with well-controlled diabetes have a better chance of escaping these serious blood vessel and nerve changes. The nurse's efforts to help the child maintain good control are very worthwhile.

School Relevance and Role of the School Nurse

Diet and Exercise

Diabetic children in school should be under careful control. They should have a regular regime of insulin, diet, and exercise. Any departures from the daily routine should raise a red flag.

The school nurse is the ideal person to correlate all of these activities, especially with the cafeteria manager and the physical education teacher, or the regular teacher in elementary schools with no organized play activities by a special teacher. These staff members need to be briefed by the nurse on their roles and the importance of diet and exercise.

The nurse should maintain frequent contact with the cafeteria manager to keep informed about any missed meals. Likewise, the teacher should be contacted just as frequently to see that the exercise level remains steady. Rainy-day activities need to be preplanned.

Monitoring of Blood and Urine Sugar

Most nurses are already familiar with paper strips to test urine sugar. The school nurse should also learn how to test blood sugar by the finger-prick technique that allows the closer control doctors are recommending. The technique is simple: the finger is pricked and a drop of blood is absorbed onto an absorbent paper strip; it is washed with water or wiped with cotton (depending on the method), and the color change is compared to a chart. The child's doctor should instruct the school nurse in proper technique, when to test, and any other concern in which the child may need help at school. The school nurse may have to be the one to initiate the partnership by offering assistance to the doctor.

Family and Physician Contact

Since juvenile diabetes is a relatively rare disease, an individual school nurse will rarely have more than two to four children to monitor at any one time. In small schools there may be none.

It is important to arrange telephone contact with more than one family member and with more than one person in the doctor's office. When diabetic children need help, they need it fast. To avoid rushing to a hospital, the school nurse needs a telephone network that is reliable and available all during the school day.

SECTION 11

COMMON CHILDHOOD RASHES

This section covers both rashes associated with internal disease, such as measles and chicken pox, and rashes not associated with internal diseases, or allergic rashes such as hives and eczema. (Note that impetigo and ringworm are discussed in Section 2.)

RASHES ASSOCIATED WITH INTERNAL DISEASE

Nature of the Disorder

Rashes associated with internal disease include those from red measles (*rubeola*), German measles (*rubella*), chicken pox, and scarlet fever. All of these conditions are contagious. The most contagious are chicken pox and red measles. The most contagious period begins one to three days before the rash appears, continues for one or two days after the rash appears, and then rapidly diminishes even though the rash may remain a day or two longer. See the chart below.

	Days of fever prior to rash	Days rash continues	Days child remains contagious after onset of fever
Red measles	2–3	5–8	4–6
German measles	0–1	1–2	2–4
Chicken pox	0–1	5–10	2–4
Scarlet fever	0–1	2–4	2–4 (if not treated)

There are many other childhood virus infections that cause various types of rashes, but most occur in children below school age. Some examples are roseola and fifth disease; all are mildly contagious.

Red measles and German measles are becoming rare because of successful immunization programs.

All of these diseases can vary in severity; the more severe cases last a little longer and remain contagious longer. Contagion does not end abruptly; the child slowly becomes less contagious. Scarlet fever is not contagious after one day of proper treatment, and if untreated, the child usually recovers spontaneously. A small percentage of children become carriers of the germ (streptococcus) while remaining in good health.

Symptoms and Brief Description

Red measles rash begins on the face, moves to the upper chest, stomach, and back, and finally to the arms. It begins as red spots about the size of a match head, and usually the spots run together. No crusts or scabs are formed. The children have red eyes, runny noses, coughs, and high fevers, and they are quite sick.

German measles begins and spreads the same way, but the rash is faint and sparse and in most cases doesn't spread much. The children usually have no symptoms other than low-grade fever and swollen lymph glands behind and below the ears. The diagnosis is often missed.

Chicken pox always begins with a tiny clear vesicle (water blister) that rapidly breaks and forms a loose crust or red scab from scratching and slight bleeding. It usually begins on the arms and legs and spreads to the trunk and face. The rash continues to erupt for two or three days, so one can see all stages of the sores at any one time—pure blisters to loose crusts.

Scarlet fever almost always begins on the face, neck, and upper chest. In more severe cases it then spreads to the trunk and arms. It starts as a diffuse reddish blush, no discrete spots, and the reddish skin feels rough to the touch, almost like gooseflesh. The child may or may not feel sick, depending on the severity of the disease. Inexperienced observers will often mistake the disease for red measles, a serious mistake because the treatment is completely different. Untreated scarlet fever can result in serious kidney or heart disease. Scarlatina and scarlet fever are exactly the same disease. Doctors occasionally use the name scarlatina for mild cases so as not to alarm patients unduly.

ALLERGIC RASHES

Nature of the Disorder

Allergic rashes are commonly seen. Impetigo and ringworm are discussed in Section 2.

Causes of Allergic Rashes

1. *Contact dermatitis.* The most common is poison ivy or oak, though there are many other plants whose contact can cause a rash in susceptible individuals. Many substances can cause contact dermatitis; fiberglass particles can make anybody's skin itch and cause a temporary rash. Some children develop allergic rashes from wool or animal fur.

2. *Food rashes.* Food allergy is well known, and rashes therefrom can take multiple forms. A physician's skills are required for diagnosis.

3. *Inhalant rashes.* Certain allergic individuals develop rashes from various dusts, pollens, or other substances.

Types of Allergic Rashes

1. *Hives (urticaria).* Hives usually appear as round or oval, pale reddish spots with slightly raised borders. They are usually the size of a dime or a quarter and occasionally come together to form irregular shapes. The spots come and go and reappear, sometimes several times in an hour or two. Occasionally, the eyelids, lips, or other parts of the body will also swell.

2. *Eczema.* This is an allergic rash usually seen in the bends of the elbows, backs of the knee joints, and cheeks. It can, however, appear almost anywhere on the body except the palms and soles. It is rough and scaly and often bleeds from scratching. It is a chronic condition, and most victims have had it for a long time.

3. *Miscellaneous allergic rashes.* There are innumerable types of allergic rashes, varying from large red splotches to scaly, pinpoint scabby sores that can spread and join into larger scabs that can last from a few minutes to many days.

Diagnosis

At times the school nurse or other personnel will be able to identify the condition with certainty; on occasion a visit to the doctor may be necessary. Rashes from completely different causes may look somewhat alike, but a physician can almost always say whether or not the rash is contagious, even if at times the cause may escape precise identification.

Treatment

While red measles, German measles, and scarlet fever need various treatments, their rash does not itch enough to require treatment. Scarlet fever can usually be completely cured with penicillin and always needs to be treated by a physician.

The rash of chicken pox only needs to be treated to relieve itching. For a small number of itchy pox, plain calamine lotion helps. For itching all over the body, an oatmeal bath is helpful. One cup of oatmeal, cooked until liquid is evaporated, wrapped in cheesecloth, and swirled in a tub of warm water, makes an excellent soaking solution to relieve itching. A baking soda bath also helps. Usc one cup of baking soda in a tubful of hot water.

For rashes not associated with internal disease, like those from impetigo, ringworm, scabies, eczema, and hives, many ointments and lotions are available. In some cases oral antihistamines are helpful. These medications should always be prescribed by a physician.

Role of the School Nurse

There are two questions the school nurse will be asked:

1. Is the condition contagious?
2. Should the child be excluded from school, and, if so, for how long?

Rashes associated with internal diseases are almost always contagious; the child should be seen by a doctor and not allowed to reenter school until the doctor says he or she is no longer contagious. Impetigo, ringworm, and scabies are also contagious.

Allergic rashes are never contagious. If the child is comfortable, he or she may safely attend school.

Some children with common childhood diseases are excluded from school longer than necessary. Each nurse should have access to a copy of the publication by the American Academy of Pediatrics entitled *Report of the Committee on Infectious Diseases*, commonly known as the Red Book. It may be obtained by writing to the Academy at P.O. Box 1034, Evanston, IL 60204. Chicken pox and mumps are the two diseases most commonly excluded for too long. Neither ever requires exclusion for more than seven days, usually less, unless complications develop.

SECTION 12

CHILD ABUSE

This section identifies the different kinds of child abuse covered by various state laws today and some of the major characteristics of home life in cases of such abuse. It also describes ways in which the school nurse can intervene to help an abused child.

NATURE OF THE DISORDER

Cruelty to children has been practiced in many cultures since the beginning of recorded history, and is even a part of the early mythology of many ancient peoples. Infanticide, commercial exploitation, and punishment for exorcism of malevolent spirits have all been extensively practiced in "civilized" as well as "less civilized" societies. The forms of child abuse commonly seen in America and Europe today, however, differ in various important ways from the practices described above.

Investigations into the type of child abuse seen in our society began in the mid-1940s with reports by radiologist John Caffey. He speculated that multiple fractures in infants and young children could have been purposefully inflicted by parents. Other reports in the medical and lay press and the involvement of social service agencies led to federal intervention. Slowly, during the 1950s and 1960s, investigations by physicians, social workers, and psychologists led to an understanding of the pathologic dynamics and interactions that are so often seen in families in which an abused or battered child is found.

There are four categories of child abuse:

1. Physical abuse
2. Sexual abuse
3. Emotional abuse
4. Child neglect

All four are dealt with by various state laws and all require reporting to the proper authorities. Definitions vary but are similar in each state. The last two categories—emotional abuse and neglect—are difficult to define, and usually only severe cases are reported.

FAMILIES WITH A POTENTIAL FOR ABUSE

1. Parents who abuse their children usually have had disastrous rearing experiences when they were children; often they themselves were beaten severely.

2. The family living in isolation is a common characteristic. There is no extended support system of relatives or friends. Even a telephone may not be available.
3. Since a normal support system was lacking most of their lives, abusive parents never learned how to ask for help or how to trust others. Learning to trust and have confidence in others begins in earliest infancy with eye contact, early touching and cuddling, and voice communication. If they experience pain instead of pleasure, unpleasantness intead of joy, it is only natural that toddlers or children would withdraw from the type of stimulation necessary to fulfill normal developmental needs. Continued behavior of this nature would produce a relatively noncommunicative, nonnurturing adult who would find it difficult to confide in others.
4. Some children are abused because they do not fulfill parental expectations. Such a child may be particularly difficult to raise because of excessive infantile colic, squirminess, or hyperactivity. An abused or neglected child is often used as a scapegoat and the whole family participates in the maltreatment.

SOCIOECONOMIC LEVEL

It is generally stated that child abuse occurs at all socioeconomic levels of our society. However, all studies of collected data show that many more cases occur among the lower classes. There are probably two explanations for this:

1. Most middle- to upper-class individuals utilize private physicians rather than hospital emergency rooms, and therefore cases are less likely to be reported.
2. Poorer parents cannot afford recreation, babysitters, and other means of relieving the stresses associated with child rearing. Also, at lower socioeconomic levels, more youthful marriages, teenage pregnancies, and illegitimate pregnancies occur.

ROLE REVERSAL

An abused, neglected, and maltreated child is often the victim of an insidious process by which parents expect the child to take on a nurturing role completely and grossly out of keeping with the child's normal developmental abilities. Some mothers, especially teenagers, have babies out of a need for someone to love them, and they expect the child to fulfill that need. Such a young mother who was herself raised in a stressful situation may lack the ability to nurture. She is apt to respond with anger and blame the baby when faced with the difficult realities of child rearing. As the years pass, this child will be expected to provide more and more support and nurture to the parent. The child, completely unable to fill these unrealistic expectations, slowly develops a deep feeling of guilt and may grow to feel that the physical abuse is deserved. Such children become protective of their parents and refuse to divulge information. As adults, they have problems in developing adequate self-esteem. Normally, children are expected to make mistakes; abused children are not allowed to make mistakes and thus develop poor decision-making abilities. They do not learn that they can control their own lives. (It is this feeling of confidence in our own abilities that gives us the ability to control our actions, even though we may not be able to control our feelings. "Getting mad at the baby is OK; hitting her is not.")

School Relevance and Role of the School Nurse

The school nurse can perform a specific role in effectively intervening on behalf of an abused child.

All bruises, burns, or other lesions should be measured, described, and recorded as to size, shape, and location. Photographs are very helpful. Any statements the child makes about the origin of the lesion should be recorded.

If sexual abuse is reported by a child, the person who received this trust should interview the child and record details. However, a physical examination should be done by a doctor, not by the school nurse.

Emotional abuse is almost never reported because its definition is so vague. This type of problem can be handled by the school counselor or principal in addition to the nurse. The home problems are usually so severe that not much can be done at school.

Neglect in school-age children may be reportable when a parent refuses to seek treatment for a child with an illness that has a real potential for serious complications. Common examples are untreated middle ear infections or serious impetigo.

Failure to bathe, dirty clothes, or other forms of poor personal hygiene, while regrettable, are not grounds for reporting a case of child neglect.

From the above description, it can readily be seen that merely caring for the injuries or neglect that a maltreated child suffers is a shortsighted approach. All 50 state legislatures now have mandatory reporting requirements. *Anyone* who suspects that a child has been seriously abused is required by law to report the case to the proper authorities. In schools, the teacher or school nurse usually reports suspected cases to the principal, who then makes the official report to the proper social, legal, or medical agency.

The school nurse is in a particularly advantageous position from which to detect abused children. Any child who does not engage in normal play, is withdrawn, or assumes a nurturing role inappropriate to his or her age should raise some suspicion. Gentle attempts at conversation may reveal a guarded attitude about parents and home. Such children should be watched, not only for the nurture they need, but also for other more overt signs of abuse or neglect.

Most states are now connected to computer networks that keep track of child-abuse cases nationwide. Since many abusive parents are very mobile and at the same time evasive about the injuries they inflict, this computerized information can be most helpful in deciding if a child injured under suspicious circumstances has previously been reported for suspected child abuse.

The school nurse obviously will have a small role in the actual treatment of injuries or specific guidance and counseling of parents. However, if the nurse has a basic understanding of the pathologic, emotional, and social processes underlying child abuse, a great deal of support can be given to a very needy child, and some guidance can be provided for school officials concerning the medical aspects of the problem.

SECTION 13

DISORDERS OF BEHAVIOR

This section covers a variety of behavior disorders that occur in children, including school refusal and phobia, speech disorders, enuresis, encopresis, childhood depression, suicide, autism, anorexia nervosa, bulimia, and sleeping in school.

SCHOOL REFUSAL AND PHOBIA

Nature of the Condition

Many children harbor unexpressed as well as overt fears about school. When the fear is so great that it causes the child to avoid going to school, it is necessary to determine the cause of the extended absence because the management of each case is highly specific.

School Refusal

A child may refuse to go to school for fear of a bully; another may feel unprepared for a test. An older child may simply regard school as irrelevant to his or her entire value system and future life.

Some children, instead of being afraid of the school setting, may be fearful of leaving home because of:

1. Jealousy of a younger sibling at home
2. Parental conflict, causing fear for the mother's safety in the child's absence
3. Fear of abandonment, especially when one parent has recently left
4. A recent death in the family, since the child may equate death with going away

Though these children need to learn more productive coping skills, this type of reaction pattern is not altogether abnormal. These reasons for truancy and absenteeism are not considered phobic.

School Phobia

Mental health specialists usually reserve the diagnosis of school phobia for those cases in which there is an abnormally close relationship between the child and the mother. Mother and child have an abnormal (neurotic) need for each other; when apart, they both suffer separation anxiety. Therefore, limiting management to the child always fails; the parents must participate and be involved equally.

The typical family situation conducive to the development of school phobia has been described as a large family with relatively few outside interests. Often, many relatives live in close physical proximity, and the child's parents are often closely involved with their parents. It is not the size of the family that is important; it is the isolation of that family group, extended or nuclear, from other community groups.

A school-phobic child who is forced to attend school can be expected to have many somatic complaints such as headache, stomach ache, and other body aches. Other symptoms are crying, whining, sulking, and running away from school.

Treatment

Management of school refusal or a school-phobic student requires cooperation from parents, the school nurse, teacher, counselor, therapist, and, most important, the school principal. The principal's support will determine the effectiveness of the school's role in therapy. He or she will need insight into the psychodynamics of the family's cultural and religious values in order to cooperate with a mental health specialist.

School phobia should be seen as a potentially serious condition, having ramifications beyond school. It affects a child's social relations as well as academic performance. If the family is left to its own devices, the child will rarely return to school.

All therapy is based on returning the child to school as soon as possible. All studies have shown that the longer a child remains out of school after the onset of symptoms, the longer treatment is necessary, sometimes taking months or years.

The following suggestions are useful in management:

1. Parents, usually the mother, will grasp at any straw to keep a phobic child at home—fear of failure, peer ridicule, or a strict teacher are among many reasons offered by the mother to rationalize keeping the child home. These mothers are particularly in need of an understanding and reassuring principal.

2. Though the first step in therapy should be a return to school, in severe cases family psychotherapy will be necessary for a few days before the return.
3. If treatment is initiated as late as fourth or fifth grade, the psychological process is usually more difficult to reverse.
4. To initiate treatment, a school person whom the child knows (teacher, nurse, counselor, or principal) will be best accepted. A suggested technique for reducing anxieties is to let the mother and child walk halfway to school and then both go home; later, they come in through the front door and return home together. This should progress by easy stages, always insisting that the child go a little bit further each day—visiting an hour in the library one day, progressing to an hour in class, and so on by small steps to all day in class.
5. Victimizing by peers should not be tolerated, as the frightened child is helpless to protect himself or herself.
6. The school clinic and school nurse may be a useful halfway point during the process of getting the child back into the classroom.

SPEECH DISORDERS

Stuttering

Children respond to their mothers' voices in the early weeks and months of life, long before they acquire an understanding of symbolic language. Receptive language ability continues to exceed expressive language ability throughout life.

Between the ages of two and four years, children have an urgent need to express themselves before they have developed the language fluency to do so. This is often called the period of dysfluency and is characterized by frequent syllabic repetition. If adults express concern about this normal phenomenon, the child is made to feel inadequate about his or her speech, causing self-conscious focus on the mechanics of speaking. This can impair the normal development of fluency and cause stuttering.

Of course, many other factors can also cause stuttering. Children who begin to stutter at age six or seven need a different therapeutic approach from what a three- or four-year-old needs. The school nurse should suggest that the older child be seen by the school psychologist as well as the speech pathologist.

Articulation Disorders

Errors of articulation may consist of distortions, substitutions, omissions, or lisps. Occasionally, a structural abnormality of the mouth, tongue, or palate can cause difficulty; often there is no demonstrable pathology. When remediation is necessary, the child must be referred to the speech pathologist. However, there are some children whose minor articulation imperfections are barely noticeable and who are always understood. In all probability, these children will never be handicapped by their slight lisps or occasional consonant omissions. Since referral to a speech pathologist is often stigmatizing, the school nurse can ask the speech pathologist to make a casual classroom visit for verification of the need for speech therapy.

Elective Mutism

A child who is shy by nature and speaks very little at home or at play may react to extra stress by the development of elective mutism (sometimes called selective mutism). This child is not being willful or obstinate; the inability to speak is an adaptive reaction to stress.

This rare condition, when seen, often occurs at school and may be first manifested in any of the elementary grades. The parents usually state that the child does speak when not in school. Often one of the parents also has a shy, retiring disposition.

Elective mutism usually causes great consternation at school; teacher, counselor, and principal vie with one another to see who can get the child to talk. This approach, of course, is counterproductive because the extra attention only serves to reinforce the gain that the child receives from remaining mute. Successful therapy requires complete cooperation from all school personnel and should always be supervised by a psychologist skilled in behavior management techniques. If a child is placed in an institution, rapid results may be achieved because of the strict control available; however, relapses are common with return to the previous environment. The goal of therapy is not merely to have the child say some words, but to react to stressful situations in a more normal manner.

Case histories of children with elective mutism, when followed over long periods of time, eventually report normal speech. However, 5 to 25 percent remain very poor communicators. How much of a handicap this is in later life depends completely on the individual's vocational choice and life style.

ENURESIS

Nature of the Condition

Urinary incontinence with soiling of clothes can occur during the day or night. Though some children are toilet trained by age three, so many children have frequent accidents up to age five that it can hardly be considered abnormal. Between the ages of three and six, whether it is considered abnormal or not depends a great deal on parental expectations. In some families, there is a great deal of parental pressure for early toilet training. If the child, for whatever reason, is not constitutionally ready, or if he or she subconsciously rebels, this parental attitude is apt to cause the child to be labeled as *enuretic.* The label itself can contribute to prolonged wetting. Another child with this same problem in a relaxed household might well become completely toilet trained, day and night, by age four or five. Most pediatricians do not consider bed wetting sufficiently abnormal to require treatment before the child is six years old.

While an occasional child with enuresis will be found to have some infection or abnormality of the urinary tract, the large majority will not. The causes of nonorganic enuresis at school are legion. Two examples are too early and too demanding toilet training, and fear of going to the school rest room.

School Relevance and Management

Almost all kindergarten and first grade teachers know that many children have "accidents," and they try to protect these children from embarrassment. By the second or third grade, however, repeated urinary soiling is rare enough to be considered abnormal, and the child should be referred to a physician.

In some cases, the amount of urine expelled is so small that it can be safely ignored if it creates no disturbance.

If the teacher feels confident that the child is not using the symptom for some secondary gain, a discreet method of having the child go to the rest room once or twice a day can be arranged.

When a child is noticeably wet and smells of urine almost every day, management should be the same as for overflow incontinence of the bladder. This happens regularly in certain diseases of the lower spinal cord such as spina bifida. (See Section 17.) The parents should provide extra clothes so the child can be helped to change clothes privately.

ENCOPRESIS

Nature of the Condition

Habitual fecal soiling occurring past the ages of five to seven is known as *encopresis*. Not only are the causes more complicated than those of enuresis, but, because of the odor, more adverse social consequences are suffered.

As in children with enuresis, children with encopresis are rarely found to have organic disease or abnormality requiring surgery or specific medication. A notable exception is chronic and severe constipation. Normally, the rectum slowly fills and, at a certain point of stretch, the nerve endings send the proper message to the brain so that the individual has a normal bowel movement. If for some reason the rectum is not evacuated at that time, the urge eventually goes away until a later time. Children who are sufficiently constipated lose the urge altogether and develop a fecal impaction, a large hard mass of stool that gathers at the lower rectum and causes obstruction. The stool above the impaction then liquefies and leaks around the impaction. (See Figure 13–1.)

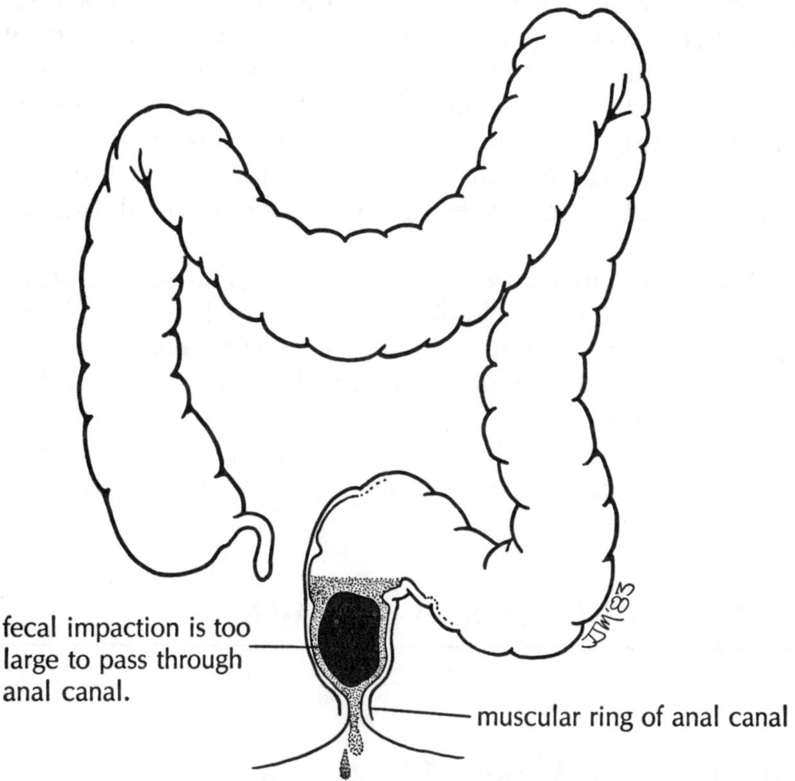

Figure 13–1. fecal impaction

Though the child is completely unaware that this is happening, the underwear is constantly soiled and the fecal odor invites derision from classmates.

Fecal soiling may also occur simply because the child will not take the time to go the bathroom. In this case, there will be a good-sized mass of stool in the pants, not the lesser amount that is seen in the overflow incontinence just described.

School Relevance and Management

These children must all be referred to a physician. A fecal impaction is easily diagnosed by a digital rectal examination. It can be removed by a gentle water or mineral oil enema, repeated two to three times if necessary, plus mineral oil given by mouth. Each child's oral dose of mineral oil is different; it should be given every night or two in an amount sufficient to cause a full-sized soft stool each day but not enough to cause leaks and stained pants. For children who dislike plain mineral oil, there are several emulsified flavored products available. After sufficient time, usually three to six months, the rectum regains its tone and rhythmicity, and bowel movements can occur normally without mineral oil.

Classroom management is similar to that of the severe enuretic. An extra set of clothes should always be on hand, and the nurse should enlist the aid of the teacher, counselor, and principal to help the child get to the bathroom with as little humiliation as possible.

Children who do not have a fecal impaction may be helped by psychological counseling or behavioral management techniques.

CHILDHOOD DEPRESSION

Nature of the Condition

All normal individuals, child and adult, feel depressed at various times in their lives. However, when mental health specialists speak of *depression,* they don't mean temporarily feeling down; they mean a distinct disease entity that strongly affects the total personality. Depression usually lasts several months or years and often requires specific medical or psychiatric treatment such as psychotherapy or psychoactive medication. There is no question that depression is one of the most common psychiatric disorders in adults. It also occurs with less frequency in children.

Classification

1. *Endogenous depression* implies that the patient has an innate or inborn psychological weakness that predisposes him or her to depression.
2. *Reactive depression* is thought to be caused by adverse environmental or situational circumstances. In school children, a suspected cause is continued classroom failure and repeated loss in most of the everyday life struggles that all children face.

Symptoms

Direct

1. Feelings of boredom, helplessness, or hopelessness
2. Loneliness, isolation, or withdrawal
3. Feelings of sadness
4. Diminished enthusiasm and physical activity
5. Self-deprecatory statements
6. Suicidal ideas, expressions, or actual attempts

Indirect or Masked

The masked symptoms are those compensatory or coping mechanisms the depressed child develops to protect his or her self-esteem:

> The wish to avoid sadness and humiliation is a powerful motivating force and a major determinant of behavior for all school-age children. If a child cannot measure up to expected school performance, he [or she] often will react with some form of socially maladaptive behavior to save face. Such a child may live with an ever-present threat of exposure and peer ridicule. Many adults also are engaged in a constant effort to avoid humiliation, but for them the task is an easier one. If they can't dance, they don't go to dances! If they are not good at reading, they can go to movies! Children, however, are required to pursue activities that display weaknesses likely to lead to humiliation. (Adapted from Levine,

Brooks, and Shonkoff's *A Pediatric Approach to Learning Disorders* (New York: John Wiley & Sons, 1980).)

Common indirect or masked symptoms are:

1. Headaches, stomach aches, or other body complaints
2. Silliness and clowning
3. Aggression, fighting, and rebelliousness
4. Poor school performance
5. Physical tiredness (often in adolescents)

Drug use is a common symptom of adolescent depression. This is often explained as being the result of fear or inability to express or discuss inner conflicts. This inability results in suppression of normal aggressive tendencies. The use of drugs makes the adolescent withdraw and feel better and thus avoid having to deal with aggression.

Long-term studies of large groups of children at various ages have been done in an attempt to determine how frequently the symptoms of masked depression occur in a normal population since most of the symptoms occur at various times in many children's lives. One study of seventh and eighth grade children (Kovacs and Beck) showed that 33 percent were depressed to a degree labeled moderately severe. Such a high incidence rate casts great doubt on the validity of the diagnosis, especially since all of the children were performing well in school. This and other studies have led some researchers to the following conclusion:

> The concept of a syndrome of masked childhood depression is as yet unsubstantiated and...a diagnosis of this condition in children would appear to be premature and treatment unwarranted. The possibility of producing iatrogenic (doctor-induced) effects on the child, the risk of masking other problems, and the unknown effects on the parents underscore the need for rigorous research of this question. (Lefkowitz and Burton, 1978.)

Treatment and School Relevance

It is impossible to generalize about the management of the so-called depressed child; treatment is largely symptomatic. However, school nurses and teachers can be guided by certain principles:

1. Never try to manage a depressed child without professional consultation from a psychologist, psychiatrist, or family doctor. Involve the counselor, principal, and parents as much as possible.
2. Depressed children are very moody and always suffer from very low self-esteem. Though it is easier for a teacher to deal with a sad, quiet six-year-old than an angry, belligerent thirteen-year-old, both need individual attention.
3. It will be impossible for a classroom teacher to take time to meet all the needs of a depressed child. It is important, however, to have some insight into the underlying problems so as not to unknowingly embarrass the child and perhaps provoke further maladaptive behavior.
4. Maladaptive behavior must not be condoned. While one cannot be overly strict in every detail, it is important for such children to know that the teacher is aware of what they are doing. Aggression, giving up too easily, poor school performance, and so on, should be confronted confidentially and directly, not glossed over.
5. Consistent, sustained academic achievement is impossible for depressed children. If they can be taught to sublimate their aggression, perform easy-to-complete tasks, relate to peers, and assume some age-appropriate responsibilities, their achievement and self-concept will also improve.
6. Drug treatment of childhood depression with adult-type, mood-elevating medication is quite controversial at this time. Some children do seem to benefit from its use, however, and a school nurse can make a real contribution to the child's therapy by observing and reporting changes in behavior.

SUICIDE

Nature of the Condition

It is helpful to think of suicidal behavior as a symptom of a medical condition that can be cured. A helpful analogy is appendicitis. If undiagnosed and untreated, the appendix ruptures and the patient dies. If properly diagnosed and treated, recovery can be expected.

Similarly, disregard of the premonitory clues preceding suicide often leads to death. Proper diagnosis and treatment can lead to a long and reasonably happy life. The suicide rate in children and adolescents is unquestionably rising. It is now the fourth leading cause of death in the teen years, ranking just behind homicide, cancer, and accidents. For many years the rate was fairly stable at about 4 per 100,000, but it is now estimated at about 16 per 100,000 in the population age 12 to 19. Moreover, the quoted figures are misleading because many accidents are actually suicides. Well-meaning physicians and coroners often certify a death as accidental rather than suicidal in suspicious circumstances, to spare the family additional grief.

Attempts are much more common; estimates range from 200 to 400 for every successful suicide. Boys succeed more often than girls because they tend to use more lethal methods, such as guns and hanging. Girls usually overdose with pills and can be resuscitated. Anglo-Saxon attempts predominate over blacks and Hispanics, but the differences are less than formerly. The incidence is higher in first-born children.

As in adolescents, the incidence of suicide and attempted suicide is also rising in children from four to twelve years of age. These young children come from the same types of homes as the older children and also feel hopeless, helpless, and abandoned. At the age of ten or twelve, children's concept of death begins to change. Before this time, they do not fully understand the finality of death, thinking of it more as "going away." As they grow older, their concept approaches that of the adult.

Abused children often come to think of themselves as bad children and attempt suicide as a response to a feeling of guilt for having caused their parents so much trouble. As they become older and better able to perceive the reality of the situation, they are more apt to have "you'll be sorry after I'm dead" feelings.

School nurses and teachers need to be alert to the same premonitory signs in younger children as in adolescents, especially in children who have "accidentally" ingested poisons. Many studies have shown that over the age of six true accidental poisoning is extremely rare. The younger children are issuing the same calls for help as are the adolescents, and they are more amenable to therapy.

Causes

Most suicides occur in children of unstable or broken homes, often a single-parent home. The children feel unloved and unwanted and develop a poor self-concept.

A suicidal child is most often depressed, with either overt symptoms or symptoms masked in the form of hostility, delinquency, or dare-devil and self-destructive behavior. Adolescents are often bored, restless, can't concentrate, rapidly lose interest in any pursuit, and seek constant activity to escape depressed feelings. They are frequently impulsive and immature and overreact even to minor stresses.

Clues

In a child with symptoms described above, danger signals that precede suicide attempts are:

1. Writing notes or poetry with themes related to death
2. Giving away prized possessions
3. Repeated serious trauma (burns or accidents)
4. Family history of suicide

School Relevance and Management

A suicide attempt or signal should always be viewed as a call for help and should always be responded to. Failure to respond simply reinforces the feelings of rejection and makes the next attempt more imminent.

The child should be referred to the school counselor, who in turn needs backup help from the school psychologist or a psychiatrist. Most children who have attempted suicide need a period of medical or psychiatric treatment at home or in a hospital. Those who are overtly psychotic always need to be seen by a psychiatrist.

If a school nurse, counselor, or teacher has established a comfortable, friendly relationship with a student, and many of the premonitory suicidal tendencies are present, it might help to ask directly about suicidal thoughts. This must be done in a tactful way, at the right time, and with due regard for privacy. Asking about suicide does not cause suicide.

AUTISM

Nature of the Condition

Autism is sometimes thought of as infantile or early childhood schizophrenia, but the differences between the autistic child and the preteen or adolescent schizophrenic are so great that the prevailing consensus is that they are separate and distinct conditions.

Originally it was believed that autism in children was largely caused by a lack of nurturing and improper parenting; it was thought to exist in the children of cold and aloof parents. However, it is now fairly universally agreed that autism is an organic developmental disability whose cause is not related to parental management.

Autism is a very strange disorder. It is relatively rare, and some school nurses, especially in the upper grades, have never seen a case. However, it would be beneficial to visit a facility for autistic children or to see a documentary film showing such children at various ages and activities.

Symptoms

1. *Aloneness.* Autistic children truly live in a world of their own. They relate to people as they relate to a table. Occasionally the child will respond to speech, but erratically, seldom, and often

inappropriately. Occasionally they will speak, but with little relationship to what is happening or what they want.

2. *Onset at an early age.* Symptoms always appear before three years of age. Occasionally, with hindsight, parents can recall that during infancy their baby would not cuddle or snuggle. As toddlers, they did not follow their parents or go to them for comfort.

3. *Delayed and deviant language development.* Fully 50 percent never gain useful speech, and those who do often use it in an abnormal fashion. There is persistent *echolalia* (echoing the words of others) of words and phrases and error in choice of pronoun (I–you). Speech is used in a noncommunicative manner—it lacks a give-and-take quality. Only the present exists; what happened earlier is never mentioned. The precursors of oral language, such as "pat-a-cake" or "bye-bye," don't develop. Speech onset is late and comprehension is very poor. There is a lack of appropriate gesture—instead of pointing with the finger, the whole hand is used; if the child wants an object, he or she will take an adult's hand and lead the adult to it rather than ask for it. Simple spoken commands by a parent or teacher require accompanying gestures for complete understanding.

4. *Grossly impaired social development with specific characteristics.*

a. Quality of aloneness described above.
b. A compulsive insistence on sameness with resistance to change. Requires same object at all times. Older children become obsessed with bus routes, colors, numbers, and so on.
c. Ritualistic behavior such as touching.
d. Lack of cooperative group play. No imaginative games. Much stereotyped and repetitive behavior.
e. No friends.
f. Lack of empathy or ability to perceive feelings of others. Often saying or doing things that are socially inappropriate.
g. Eye contact deficient and abnormal. "Even when he looks at me, he doesn't seem to be seeing me."
h. Occasional exceptional rote memory.

Relationship to Mental Retardation

Skillful testing has revealed that autistic children vary greatly in their intellectual capacity and that IQ scores are good predictors of educational attainments. Also, it appears that IQ scores remain stable over long periods of time. Thus, it is felt that an autistic child with a very low IQ score is just as retarded as a nonautistic child with a very low IQ score. Autism and mental retardation may coexist.

Most autistic children have a normal physical appearance, but those with concomitant mental retardation may have the facial features commonly seen in nonautistic retarded children. Also, autistics with a phenomenal rote memory will usually have a high IQ.

Those with lower IQ scores are apt to be less socially competent; they are prone to exhibit more bizarre behavior (inflict self-injury, smell other people, etc.).

Organic Brain Damage

As yet, no specific, localized brain damage that is consistent for all autistics has been found. A sizeable proportion of autistic children develop such neurologic abnormalities as epilepsy in later life, especially those with lower IQ scores.

As stated earlier, the consensus is that there is some undetected anatomical or chemical brain abnormality.

Prognosis

Much depends on the intellectual level. If the IQ score is over 70, about 75 percent gain competency in basic arithmetic skills and go on to more education or find paid employment. If the IQ score is below 70, the figure is only 20 percent.

The overall prognosis for the autistic child is generally unfavorable; most eventually reside in institutions. To keep an older autistic child at home requires special physical and caretaking facilities that most parents do not have. An autistic child with superior intellectual capacity will be educable, and extra efforts in his or her behalf are well worth the extra time and energy required.

Treatment and School Relevance

As can be imagined, many and various treatments, rational and irrational, have been tried. None has succeeded with any consistency. Occasionally a case is reported to have improved with vitamins, minerals, manipulations, and so on. Naturally, a parent will not stop using any irrational treatment if it appears to be helping, so unless it is actually harmful it is usually best to adopt a wait-and-see attitude.

The only "therapy" that consistently yields good results is proper behavior modification, often requiring strong aversive methods. This type of therapy only modifies symptoms but is quite effective and especially necessary to control self-destructive actions such as severe head banging or biting.

Classroom management is extremely difficult. Most often a special facility is required, but if a teacher has an autistic child in class, that teacher has every right to demand expert professional assistance and consultation. Through medical or psychiatric contacts, the school nurse can help in this liaison.

Parents of these children are equally in need of help. Their greatest need is to be able to get away at frequent intervals. In many large cities, respite care facilities are available, but if not, private-duty nurses or tranquilizing medications may be necessary. Parent self-help organizations are very helpful, and the school nurse can help the parents locate them. Since the passage of P.L. 94–142, more school districts throughout the United States have developed special facilities for autistic children.

ANOREXIA NERVOSA

Nature of the Condition

Anorexia nervosa can be described as a relentless pursuit of excessive thinness. It is not a dislike of food, simply a pathological desire to be always thinner and thinner. Patients are obsessed with food, they enjoy preparing it for others, and they frequently work at food-related jobs, such as waiting on tables. They collect large numbers of diet cookbooks. When they do eat, they often cut their food up into tiny pieces and chew each one slowly so that a meal may last an inordinately long time.

At first, the dieting is mild and intentional, and the patient receives approval. However, the sinister nature of the disease slowly manifests itself, and losing weight becomes an obsession; no matter how thin they become, the patients always want to be thinner. Finally, after sufficient weight loss, symptoms of starvation such as debility, fatigue, and clouding of consciousness begin to take their toll.

Symptoms

Ninety to 95 percent of patients are girls between 15 and 19 years of age who were never overweight to any remarkable degree. The condition sometimes begins as young as 11 years and as old as 40 years. By the time the patients come to medical attention they are shockingly thin. As long ago as 1689, a Dr. Richard Martin described a patient: "I do not remember that I did ever in all my practice see one...so much wasted...(like a skeleton only clad with skin) yet there was no fever but on the contrary a coldness of the whole body."

There is always intense family involvement and interaction. At first the parents merely tell their daughter that she is thin enough but they soon discover that she wants to be forever thinner. Sometimes they force the child to eat but this often leads to induced vomiting, either openly or secretly. The disease may have existed for quite some time before the parents are even aware of it because at this age parents often don't see their children undressed, and the facial fat pads don't disappear until late in the process of starvation.

The daily calorie intake becomes an obsession. A girl who has put herself on a diet of 800 calories per day (already dangerously low) may cut it down to 400 calories per day "just to be sure."

Vomiting, spontaneously or with the help of a finger or spoon down the throat, is a dangerous complication. Some anorexic patients develop bulimia and vomit after a binge of rapid, excessive eating.

Excessive laxatives and diuretics may be used along with induced vomiting. The laxative excess causes burning and pain in the stomach with intestinal cramps. In addition, there is a dangerous loss of minerals, particularly sodium and potassium. Patients who vomit and overuse laxatives and diuretics are in particular danger, and it is in this group of young girls that fatalities may occur.

Exercise excess as a method of burning up calories often occurs in the form of bicycling, running, swimming, and calisthenics. As patients get thinner, they exercise even more.

Mirror gazing occasionally occurs. Patients will stand nude in front of a mirror for long periods of time, taking satisfaction from their thinness, though they may be a mere "bag of bones." This is considered a poor prognostic sign.

Amenorrhea (cessation of menstruation) eventually occurs in all anorexic girls, but in about half of the cases the menstrual periods stop at about the same time as the dieting begins. It is known that prolonged starvation causes cessation of menstruation (as in women in prisoner-of-war camps); therefore, it was first thought that the amenorrhea of anorexia nervosa was caused only by the severe weight loss. Since about half of the patients stop menstruating before they lose any appreciable weight, it is postulated that there may be some primary disturbance in the hypothalamus, a part of the brain that controls appetite and also, to some extent, menstruation. The significance of this dilemma remains undecided.

Stealing is seen in some patients, usually food at first in binge eaters, and then money to buy food. Later they may begin stealing trinkets or jewelry to wear for adornment. The stealing has a compulsive quality to it and usually stops after successful treatment of the anorexia nervosa.

The typical patient comes to the doctor about one to two years after dieting, vomiting or purging, and beginning of excessive exercises and family disruption. They usually have lost about 20 to 40 percent of their ideal body weight and are very emaciated, but they do not think of themselves as being excessively thin. They have a characteristic life style that derives satisfaction only from the denial of calories and refusal of outside help from parents, physicians, or other health professionals. When they do finally go to the doctor, they reject any suggestions that they should increase their caloric intake.

Psychological Profile

Girls with anorexia nervosa are usually of a compulsive nature. They maintain a neat appearance and are concerned about proper clothing and grooming. They usually get good grades in school, often higher than one would expect from their IQ tests. However, they seem to be joyless individuals and derive little satifaction from their good grades. They often have strong feelings of helplessness and unworthiness with a paralyzing sense of ineffectiveness. Parents often describe their daughter as the perfect child. Adjectives commonly used to describe her are cooperative, obedient, intelligent, thoughtful, considerate, and even-tempered; "she's the last one who would have caused trouble."

Diagnosis

The diagnostic criteria are as follows:

1. Fear of obesity becoming worse as the patient gets thinner
2. Disturbance of body image, feeling fat even when thin
3. Loss of at least 25 percent of original body weight
4. Refusal to maintain body weight over minimum normal weight for age and height
5. No other physical or mental illness that accounts for weight loss
6. Amenorrhea (eventually seen in almost all patients)

Treatment

The earlier the disease is recognized and treatment is begun, the better are the chances for cure. Most established cases require a period of separation from the family, usually in a hospital.

Treatment must be both psychologically and medically oriented. Strict behavior modification with clearly defined goals (such as one to three pounds of weight gain per week) is the method usually employed today. The diet must be carefully selected so it will be acceptable to the patient and will also restore minerals, vitamins, and all other nutrients. Only rare severe cases require tube feeding and intravenous feeding.

Prognosis

Considering all types of cases from mild to severe, the long-term outlook is not particularly favorable. The usual figures quoted are about as follows:

Good outcome—40 percent
Intermediate outcome—30 percent
Poor outcome—25 percent

The mortality rate is 2 to 5 percent. Death is usually caused by an infection (such as pneumonia) at a time when all of the body resources are so depleted that all resistance is gone and no antibodies can be manufactured to fight the disease.

In the 70 percent of patients who recover, most remain preoccupied with diet and weight for many years. Recurrences are common. Only about 20 to 25 percent of all cases return to perfectly normal health.

A poor prognosis can be guessed at if the following factors exist: long duration, lower weight at beginning of treatment, unsuccessful past treatment, vomiting, and excess use of laxatives and diuretics.

School Relevance and Role of the School Nurse

Since most cases begin in girls of high school age, school personnel can play a large part in early diagnosis and can also assist in treatment. Those most involved will be the school nurse, the counselor or principal, and the physical education teacher.

The school nurse is in a position to integrate the efforts of the parents, school personnel, and physician. Any girl who shows the two most outstanding symptoms—sadness or solitude and weight loss—should be watched for a time to see if initial suspicions are confirmed. The physical education teacher should be consulted to see if the girl resists "suiting up" and, if she does, if she is unusually thin. If necessary, the student can be asked to come to the clinic weekly or monthly to be weighed. Since this is usually a growth period, any sustained weight loss should raise a red flag and the other symptoms can be looked for.

Parents usually discover the disease quite late in its course, and since the prognosis is better with an early diagnosis school personnel can play a key role. All that is required is an awareness of the disease and a relatively high index of suspicion.

Once the diagnosis is established, the school nurse can integrate and support the parents' and physician's efforts. The counselor and physical education teacher can be enlisted to form a team that is actively supportive and thus assist in producing a favorable outcome.

There are two concrete steps the school nurse can take to help in therapy:

1. Weekly or monthly weighing with support and encouragement
2. Letting the patient use the school clinic as a refuge (girls with anorexia, being somewhat depressed and feeling helpless, need support from as many sources as possible)

BULIMIA

Pure *bulimia* consists of episodic and uncontrollable urges to eat excessively and an inability to stop. These episodes are called binges. The food chosen is usually sweet, highly caloric, and capable of being eaten rapidly with little chewing. Binge eating usually occurs in solitude and may stop if interrupted by someone. When the binge is over, patients may go to sleep or vomit, either spontaneously or by insertion of a finger or spoon in the back of the throat.

While eating, the binges are pleasurable but the patient experiences post-binge anguish and depressed mood.

When not combined with anorexia, the weight varies, but patients usually do not lose and gain excessively and the weight losses are never so extreme as to be life-threatening or incapacitating; however, bulimia occurs more often as a complication of anorexia nervosa.

Anorexia nervosa and bulimia are two separate conditions; however, they may coexist in the same person, usually an older adolescent or young adult. Anorexia nervosa consists of a preoccupation with being thin; individuals suffering from it become thin to the point of emaciation. Bulimia consists of uncontrollable binge eating, usually of soft starchy foods that require little chewing. After the binge, patients often vomit or fall asleep. These patients are usually near normal weight.

When the two disorders occur together, the bulimia exists as a complication of the anorexia and the patient appears as a typical anorexic, thin to the point of emaciation.

SLEEPING IN SCHOOL

Nature of the Condition

There are three reasons why children fall asleep in school:

1. In a home in which children are permitted to stay awake much too late, having to awaken around 6:00 or 7:00 A.M. to get to school on time leaves them lacking sufficient sleep to satisfy the developmental needs for their age. They get sleepy during the day, usually right after lunch but sometimes even before noon. The amount of drowsiness varies from not paying attention to nodding, putting their heads down on their desks, and falling sound asleep.

2. Some children fall asleep as a reaction to stress. This bizarre emotional reaction has been reported in adults on the battlefield during actual combat. (A child's most frequent reaction to stress is stomach ache or headache.) Stress-induced sleep is seen

in children who are unhappy in school because of poor academic achievement or poor social adjustment.

3. *Narcolepsy* is an organic disorder somewhat related to epilepsy. True narcolepsy is very rare.

Diagnosis

Insufficient Sleep

1. Home visits to interview family members, sometimes not during school hours, are often necessary. One may find that the child stays awake till 11:00 or 12:00 midnight, occasionally till 1:00 or 2:00 A.M.
2. The child usually falls asleep at about the same time each day.
3. Mental and emotional health is usually normal in other aspects.
4. Most children in this category will be below the third grade.

Emotional Reaction

1. Home visits and other history will reveal sufficient sleep at home.
2. The child will fall asleep at a time when he or she is under stress. It may be in the classroom during arithmetic (if that is his or her worst subject) or on the playground if he or she has no friends.
3. It may occur at any age but usually in grades three to five.
4. It may occur after school or on weekends.

Narcolepsy

1. The child will fall asleep quite suddenly while doing something interesting.
2. It may occur while sitting or standing, but rarely will falling to the ground with injury occur as in a true epileptic attack.

3. Each attack lasts about the same length of time.
4. After awakening, the child is drowsy only for a short time.
5. Medical exam often shows an abnormal brain wave pattern.
6. Academic achievement and social adaptation is normal unless there are additional cognitive and/or emotional problems.

Treatment

The underlying cause will naturally suggest the proper treatment and management.

Medical treatment is limited to medication and, as this will be helpful in only a small percentage of cases, is rarely used.

Educational management consists of special classes, lessening educational demands, and occasionally tutoring. If the home situation is completely chaotic and nothing can be done to change it, some principals have found a quiet area where a kindergartener or first grader can take a one- or two-hour nap after lunch.

Emotional support can be provided by the school nurse, counselor, or teacher. This is always an important addition to any other method of management, and often helps obtain good results.

Role of the School Nurse

1. Home visits (this is one of the most important diagnostic steps; information gathered will be most helpful)
2. Consultation with parents
3. Referral to physician
4. Liaison between parents, physician, and school personnel
5. Monitoring and/or administering medication in those rare cases when it is prescribed for narcolepsy or emotional problems

SECTION 14

PSYCHOACTIVE MEDICATIONS COMMONLY USED IN SCHOOLS

This section provides supplemental information on the different psychoactive medications commonly prescribed by physicians in the treatment of behavioral disorders and the favorable and adverse side effects caused by these medications.

All of the drugs described in this chapter require a physician's prescription. They all have multiple adverse side effects. Whoever is in charge of monitoring these medications should have ready access to the *Physician's Desk Reference* (PDR), published by Medical Economics, Oradell, N.J.

The drugs described are only the ones most commonly used. Many more are available and occasionally used by some physicians.

In this chapter the words *drugs* and *medication* are used synonymously. A psychoactive drug is one that is designed to have a primary effect on brain functioning. Many of these drugs are prescribed for children in school and are designed to have their effects during school hours. Two examples are Mellaril and Ritalin. They are used to treat children with severe behavior disorders that require medication for their control.

Examples of nonpsychoactive drugs are penicillin and reserpine (for high blood pressure).

Many drugs may have psychoactive side effects. For example, Dramamine, used for sea-sickness, on occasion makes a person sleepy though it is not classified as a psychoactive drug.

AMPHETAMINES

Ritalin (generic name methylphenidate)
Cylert (generic name pemoline)
Dexedrine (generic name dextro amphetamine)

Amphetamines are prescribed legitimately for only three conditions:

1. Hyperactivity (now called attentional deficit disorder).
2. Narcolepsy.
3. Obesity. While some doctors still use these drugs for obesity, it is considered inappropriate by most authorities.

The use of amphetamines for these last two conditions will not be discussed in this chapter.

Desirable Effects

1. Decreased motor activity, impulsivity, and distractibility.
2. Increased attention span.

Undesirable Effects

1. Loss of appetite and poor weight gain. Unless severe, nothing needs to be done; the child will regain weight during summer vacation when medication is not given.
2. Nausea, stomach ache, or headache.
3. Increased motor activity.
4. Frequent crying spells with little provocation.
5. Drowsiness.

Treatment of the above side effects consists of giving the medication after a meal, reducing the dose, or changing to a different form of amphetamine. If none of this relieves the undesirable symptoms, the medication may need to be stopped altogether.

6. Zombie-like state. This is very rare. Treatment always consists of reducing the dose or changing the medication.
7. Tics. Whether or not tics can be caused or aggravated by amphetamines is controversial. As long as the possibility exists, the school nurse must be watchful and report any new tics or worsening of old ones to the parent and/or doctor.
8. Addiction. This never occurs as long as the drug is given in small controlled doses.

Some of the amphetamines are long-acting; one dose given in the morning lasts all day. These are Dexedrine spansules, Cylert, and Ritalin–SR (sustained release). My preference is to start treatment with the short-acting drug to establish a baseline dose and to determine individual tolerance. The short-acting amphetamines usually require a morning dose between 7:00 and 8:00 A.M. and another dose between 11:00 A.M. and 12:00 noon. By the time the child gets home from school, the effects are over. Occasionally a child is so hyperactive that a third dose at about 3:00 or 4:00 P.M. will be necessary.

PHENOTHIAZINES

Thorazine (generic name chlorpromazine)
Stelazine (generic name trifluoperazine)
Mellaril (generic name thioridazine)

These drugs are often called the major tranquilizers in contrast to minor tranquilizers such as Valium and Librium. They are major because they produce more profound effects and are usually used for more serious conditions.

Their most common use in school children is for those whose behavior disorders are manifested by hostility, physical aggression, and violence.

Mellaril is occasionally used for hyperactivity if amphetamines do not help or cause serious undesirable side effects.

Desirable Effects

1. Decreased aggression and violence.
2. Decreased motor activity.

Undesirable Effects

1. Drowsiness and dryness of the mouth. These are expected effects and usually disappear in two or three weeks. If they persist or become severe, the dose may have to be reduced or the drug changed.
2. Weight gain, sluggish mood, and slow, foggy thinking.

These effects are usually dose-related; the larger the dose, the more likely they are to occur. Unfortunately, the dose required to control unacceptable behavior may in some cases cause all three undesirable side effects.

3. Further undesirable reactions. There are more than two pages of fine print in the PDR describing possible adverse side effects; some are very serious and occasionally permanent. Therefore, use of these medications requires careful

consideration. Any child receiving them must be monitored closely.

Fortunately, in the low doses usually prescribed for behavior problems in children attending school, serious reactions are rare. Serious adverse side effects are more often seen in emotionally disturbed hospitalized patients who receive much higher doses.

ANTIDEPRESSANTS

Tofranil (generic name imipramine)
Norpramin (generic name desipramine)
Elavil (generic name amitryptyline)

These drugs are used primarily to treat depression in adults, much less commonly in children. Tofranil is also used to treat bed wetting in children, but in the small doses used it is not supposed to have any psychoactive effects.

Desirable Effects

1. Elevation of mood.

Undesirable Effects

1. Dryness of mouth.
2. Sluggish mood and loss of fine motor control.
3. Further side effects. The PDR lists about as many serious side effects of the tricyclic antidepressant drugs as it does for the major tranquilizers (phenothiazines); therefore, the same warnings and instructions apply.

BENZODIAZEPINES

Librium (generic name chlordiazepoxide)
Valium (generic name diazepam)

These minor tranquilizers are usually called antianxiety drugs and are used for relief of tension. They are not helpful in children with hyperactivity or aggressive behavior disturbances.

Desirable Effects

1. Relief of tension.
2. General calming of mood.

Undesirable Effects

1. Excessive drowsiness.

These drugs are very widely used in adults, much less so in children. The occurrence of serious side effects is very rare; however, psychological addiction can occur quite easily, and they should be used only when absolutely necessary.

Drowsiness is treated by reducing the dose and, if necessary, raising it very gradually in subsequent weeks.

ROLE OF THE SCHOOL NURSE

The school nurse should record each dose of medication given at school on a chart. If the nurse is not at the school every day, the person who is delegated to give the medication should be instructed in the proper way and should record the dose on the chart. Alert school personnel about children holding pills in their mouths and later spitting them out.

When possible, arrange for all of the medication to be given at home. The phenothiazene drugs have a longer duration of action and are more amenable to this mode of administration. Also, the long-acting amphetamines may be useful.

Take care that a child who is receiving legally prescribed medication is not mistaken for a drug abuser. Because of adverse side effects, a child may appear to behave strangely or be drowsy or "stoned." In this regard, some psychotic (insane) or near psychotic children will exhibit strange, weird behavior and be suspected of drug abuse while not taking any drugs at all.

Insist that a copy of the PDR be available for the nurse and other school personnel. The nurse acts as liaison between parent, child, and physician so that undesirable side effects or lack of therapeutic effects are promptly reported.

SECTION 15

DISORDERS OF LEARNING

This section focuses on the medically related aspects of the problems of hyperactivity, dyslexia, aphasia–dysphasia, perceptual disorders, and minimal brain dysfunction; the various methods used for remediation; and the school nurse's role in the treatment of these problems.

Although untold numbers of authorities have described and defined "learning disability," there is still much disagreement. Much of what had been accepted as gospel in earlier years has been either completely discarded or is highly suspect today. The same fate will ultimately befall the truisms of today. There are many different categories of specialists who deal with this problem, and they often differ radically. Whenever controversy exists in any field—history, science, or education—one can be sure that nobody has the true answer, or more likely that there is no single answer. To illustrate, there is absolutely no argument concerning the best single medicine for a strep throat; penicillin is the undisputed choice. Entire sections of the library are filled with books and magazine articles on learning disability. I am only going to summarize those aspects of the problems that I know from personal experience are medically related.

Doctors first encounter the learning disabled child when a parent brings the child in for help. Since few doctors have had training in this subject, all too often the parent will be told there is nothing wrong. It is obvious that something is wrong when a bright child, from a normal home with normal vision and hearing, can't succeed in school. The school nurse or teacher should never accept this answer from a doctor. The parents should be urged to get further consultation from a physician specialist or child psychologist knowledgeable about these matters. There is rarely need at this stage to consult a child psychiatrist.

HYPERACTIVITY OR ATTENTIONAL DEFICIT DISORDER

Nature of the Condition

Aspects of this complex subject will be selected that are medically related and of interest to the school nurse. For further study, several good books are recommended in the bibliography.

Symptoms

Of all types of learning disabilities, hyperactivity is undoubtedly the most common. Because the most significant symptom is a deficit in attention, the official nomenclature has been changed to the *attentional deficit disorder,* or *ADD*. However, it is still popularly referred to as hyperactivity.

The primary characteristics are as follows:

1. Short attention span
2. Motor hyperactivity
3. Distractibility
4. Impulsive behavior
5. Rapid fatigue when concentration is required
6. Inability to follow a task through to its finish
7. Poor memory and learning ability

The secondary characteristics develop as a result of psychological complications:

1. Poor self-esteem; childhood depression
2. Anxiety neuroses
3. Juvenile delinquency
4. Alcoholism in adults

It occurs most often in boys and has some very distinctive features, but it is rare that any one child will exhibit all of these features. For example, some children with distinct ADD have a good memory and learning ability and grow up emotionally healthy. Some experts think they can recognize these infants by age one, but the younger the child, the more speculative the diagnosis. It is rare that preschool children need medication, but on occasion it may be necessary.

Attention deficit disorder without hyperactivity is occasionally seen. This is much harder to diagnose, because the most noticeable symptom is absent. Children with emotional problems or hearing problems, for example, may appear to have an attentional problem. Their treatment, of course, is entirely different.

Some children with ADD are born with certain innate personality characteristics that interfere with their social adjustment and lead to further maladaptive behavior. Most long-term follow-up studies reveal that children usually get over their hyperactivity by the fifth or sixth grade, but their attentional deficits may remain, they sometimes are poor readers, and they often make poor social adjustments. However, if the child is lucky enough to have good parental, medical, and educational support, he or she has an excellent chance to make it through the educational system and become a normal, successful adult.

Treatment

The usual medical approach in the United States is treatment with amphetamines, and the one most often prescribed is Ritalin. There is much controversy about the use of this type of drug. It has its ardent proponents and those dead set against it. I know from personal experience that school personnel who are opposed to amphetamine therapy prove to be right about as often as they are wrong. Amazingly enough, doctors do no better predicting which child will benefit. For the past 10 to 15 years, many researchers have been developing tests to try to predict which children will improve with amphetamines. However, the present state of the art is such that the most reliable diagnosis can be made using all or part of a multidisciplinary team of teacher, doctor, school nurse, and psychologist. A carefully monitored clinical trial will prove the effectiveness of medication. When children are handled in this manner, the results are usually conclusive in a short time. It is most important to have a built-in monitoring system so dosage can be adjusted or medication stopped if undesirable side effects or treatment failures are evidenced. Amphetamines control hyperactivity very well in about 60 percent of the cases and moderately well in another 20 percent. The remaining 20 percent are either unimproved or get worse.

Dosage, of course, must be left up to the prescribing physician. Undesirable side effects are usually not seen until the total daily dose approaches or exceeds 60 milligrams of Ritalin or 30 milligrams of Dexedrine for a five- to seven-year-old child.

It is wise never to treat ADD with medication alone. Classroom management is just as important. When a decision has been made to treat a hyperactive child with medication, it is helpful for the teacher to consider certain behavior modification techniques and minor alterations in instructional methods. Following is a list of guidelines from *A Pediatric Approach to Learning Disorders* by M. L. Levine, M.D.

1. Begin and end each day with praise for the child. Many children with attention deficits have significantly diminished self-image and feel as if there is no chance for success in school.
2. Break up work into small units. Avoid lengthy instructions and assignments whose persistence far exceeds the child's demonstrated working capacity.
3. Have a secret way of signaling a child who is inattentive to the task at hand. It is not helpful to call on a chronically inattentive child who is caught staring out the window. This may be humiliating and is likely to increase anxiety, which will further drain attention.
4. Whenever possible, such children should be in small classrooms, and the teacher should try to offer individual attention. There should be an awareness that such children may learn more on a one-to-one basis in ten minutes than they do during two hours in a large classroom.
5. A minimum of background noise and visual stimulation is helpful. A classroom with 200 different pictures on the wall, a fish tank, a gerbil cage, four terrariums, and a multicolored mobile may offer more sensory data than an inattentive child can filter.
6. Following a consistent schedule can help provide organization for such a child. Children with attention deficits generally do not adapt well to major shifts in program content or order.
7. The teacher needs to be sensitive to peer abuse. Such children sometimes have associated social ineptitudes (excess silliness, grimacing, body posturing, or "coming on too strong" when approaching a new situation or new group of friends) that cause rejection by their peers. The impact can be minimized by helping the vulnerable child to save face.
8. Motivation can be increased by involving the student in a personal way. Puzzles, finding mistakes in other people's work, and games of concentration might be tried. The

child should be helped to plan his or her work through a dialogue with the teacher or other problem-solving strategies.

9. Regular meetings with the child to discuss behavioral and academic progress are important. Offer concrete methods for feedback and monitoring (for example, graphs, scoring systems, diaries).
10. After an understanding is reached between teacher and child with regard to the attention deficit, discussion should center around whether or not the child was "tuned in" or in control of his or her attention rather than whether he or she was "bad" or "good." The concern here is that if a child is called bad often enough, this will constitute a self-fulfilling prophecy!

Because of the many articles published in the lay press about the horrible effects of medication, many classroom teachers have strong prejudices against the use of any drug for any child with behavior or learning problems. While these teachers are undoubtedly well intentioned, they are doing many children a disservice. True, the teacher knows the child well from daily observation and may well question the diagnosis and argue the case directly with the others involved, but one should never undermine the parents' confidence in these professionals through individual objections. The hyperactive child who responds well to a relatively small dose of amphetamine is being aided in a manner similar to that of a child with diabetes who receives insulin. While the medication does not cure this child, it certainly enables him or her to lead a more normal life.

DYSLEXIA

Nature of the Disorder

Dyslexia was described in the closing years of the last century by a British ophthalmologist. The word derives from the Greek *dys* ("abnormal") and *lexia* ("words" or "reading"). It was thought to be a separate entity because the child (or adult) seemed perfectly normal and bright otherwise. Factors such as hyperactivity, mental retardation, emotional disturbance, poor home environment, and lack of educational opportunity could be ruled out by tests or actual observation. At that time, experts were pretty much in agreement about who did and who did not have dyslexia.

Today, confusion reigns because all categories of experts insist on their own definitions. No one can fully agree, and some say there is no such thing as dyslexia. The National Advisory Committee on Dyslexia concluded that in view of the wide divergence of interpretation, the use of the term served no useful purpose (cited by Lerner in 1976). Any population of reading-deficient children (or adults) rarely shows similar etiology or clinical manifestations, as one would expect it would if this were any single condition.

In the confusion that has existed, various experts have postulated that individuals with dyslexia actually see words backwards (*was/saw, dog/god*). However, articulate, intelligent dyslexic adults report that their difficulty does not lie in the actual perception or "seeing" of the word or letter but in what their brain does with it after they see it. They speak of difficulty in following a line of print, finishing the end of one line, dropping down one space and beginning the next, keeping their place with small print, and so on. It is becoming increasingly evident that dyslexia is one of the many intracerebral processing deficits; not a deficit in seeing but rather associating what is seen with the proper brain connections, resulting in the ability to read and write smoothly, easily, and rapidly.

Diagnosis

In my experience in reviewing cases, observing children, and talking to teachers, the following conclusions seem likely:

1. There is an entity that can be called dyslexia.
2. It is quite rare.
3. It is a different type of disorder from the attentional deficit disorder (hyperactivity) and requires different management.

4. A child who has moderate to severe and fairly obvious emotional disturbances, hyperactivity, deranged psychosocial situations, and/or lack of educational opportunities should not be diagnosed as dyslexic.
5. Dyslexia can occur in combination with the above problems.
6. The diagnosis should be reserved for those for whom it was intended in the first place—children who are obviously of average or above average intellectual capacity and who, at the age of eight to ten years, after adequate educational opportunity, still can hardly read and are usually very poor spellers and writers. It is in this group of individuals—child and adult—that, with appropriate testing, one can diagnose true dyslexics.

Many children six to ten years of age are poor readers, sometimes to a severe degree, because they have emotional disturbances, hyperactivity, or poor psychosocial environments. Many parents of retarded or emotionally disturbed children prefer the more socially acceptable diagnosis of dyslexia for their children.

APHASIA–DYSPHASIA

Classical *aphasia* results from a cerebral hemorrhage (stroke) that destroys certain parts of the left temporal lobe of the brain—the language area. This causes the patient to lose the ability to speak, even though all of the functions associated with speech remain intact. Breath control, tongue and mouth movements, swallowing, and all of the other things we always do automatically and unthinkingly each and every time we speak, remain normal. Because the hemorrhage rarely limits itself to a tiny, exact brain area (there are no walls or membranes to hold back the blood), there is almost always destruction of surrounding brain tissue also, so frequently there are associated symptoms as well, such as difficulty in comprehension of speech and impaired writing skills. Neurologists usually think of aphasia as the loss of previously acquired normal speech.

The term *developmental dysphasia* implies that the pathology in the language area of the brain was present at birth or acquired by some unknown means in the early months of life, and *dysphasia* means a mild form of aphasia. To date there are no known tests to demonstrate whether or not these children have left temporal lobe pathology. It is logical to guess, however, that when techniques do become available, some form of brain abnormality will be found.

Dysphasic children do not develop normal speech, and their problems are quite different from those of an adult with classical aphasia. Remediation procedures, therefore, must consider this difference.

Before diagnosing developmental dysphasia, it is important to rule out other primary disorders that may cause disordered speech, such as moderately profound hearing loss (past or present), cleft palate, or mental retardation.

PERCEPTUAL DISORDERS

Dictionaries define *perception* as "the act or faculty of apprehending by means of the senses or of the mind; cognition; understanding." The verb is "to perceive" and the adjective is "perceptual." They all mean the same thing. In educational circles, however, the phrase *perceptual disorder* is used differently. Neurologists would substitute the phrase *cerebral processing disorder.*

Neurophysiologists speak of sensory nerve activity by which messages enter the brain through one of the sense organs (eyes, ears, nose, tongue, and touch) and motor nerve activity by which messages exit from the brain to direct muscle contraction or relaxation, thereby causing body movement. When the brain receives the sensory message, it calls into play large areas involving memory, intuition, feeling, opposing messages, and many other factors. It then automatically correlates and computes this multitude of input in order to send out the proper instructions so that the body will respond in an appropriate fashion to the original input message. The cerebral activity between reception and response is known as intracerebral processing. It is a most crucial and important part of brain activity. When this particular function does not work right, an individual is said to have a cerebral processing disorder. A perceptual disorder and a cerebral processing disorder are exactly the same thing. The disorder is not in how one perceives but rather in how the circuit connections of the brain computer have failed to work properly and in the usual fashion.

Educators and educational psychologists speak of various types of perceptual disorders. A *visual–motor* perceptual disorder is usually taken to mean poor eye–hand coordination, which causes poor copying ability, handwriting, and drawing. *Perceptual–motor* disorders refer to children who have poor gross and/or fine motor control and poor body coordination. Gross motor movement means moving the body or limbs through space. Fine motor movement refers to using the hands and fingers. *Auditory perceptual* and *visual perceptual* disorders have also been described. For each labeled perceptual disorder, various tests have been devised to diagnose the disorder and various exercises constructed to treat it. About ten years ago, these tests and remediation exercises were very popular and are still used by some with faith in their reliability. However, research and clinical experience have cast doubts on the effectiveness of tests that purport to diagnose these disorders and the exercises that are supposed to remediate them. Children with perceptual disorders undoubtedly have impaired learning ability, but just exactly which cerebral process is impaired is not known. At present, some of the specific processes being studied are sequencing ability, spatial arrangement ability, memory (both long- and short-term), and attention span. Neurologists are not even sure what part or parts of the brain control these functions.

In light of what is known after years of observations, most educators, pediatricians, and neurologists feel that the best measures to remediate perceptual handicaps are not by perceptual exercises but by dealing directly with the educational deficiencies through various special educational techniques. Some students need to postpone studying those subjects that cause undue frustration or emotional problems. The entire subject of educational remediation is very complex. Certain aspects of it will be dealt with in the section on remediation below.

MINIMAL BRAIN DYSFUNCTION

At the present time, the term *MBD*—for *minimal brain dysfunction*—is rarely used. There have been many recent advances in diagnosis and categorization of the various types of learning disorders, perceptual disorders, attentional deficits, and so on. Therefore, the term MBD has been largely discarded in favor of the specific entity that differs from child to child. Often this entity can be diagnosed with specificity for each child. Some of the specific entities are disorders of sequencing, memory, spatial or temporal arrangement, and attention.

However, MBD is so firmly entrenched in professional literature that an understanding of what it means is essential. Until the late 1950s, the predominant opinion was that if a child had normal intelligence and didn't learn, he or she had psychological problems. Toward the end of the decade, a prominent pediatric textbook added a new section entitled "Behavior Problems Associated with Organic Brain Damage." Children with short attention span, distractibility, impulsiveness, various perceptual difficulties, and several other symptoms were included under this heading. This set the stage for the decade of the 1960s, when organic–biological factors rated equally important with emotional–psychological factors as a cause of learning disability.

In about 1962, lacking conclusive evidence of actual brain damage, the concept of brain "dysfunction" was introduced, and though the initials remained the same the majority of experts began to use the term *minimal brain dysfunction* to describe the constellation of symptoms formerly described as minimal brain damage. During this decade, various educational, psychological, and medical experts developed the 50 or 60 names alluded to below, resulting in a jumble of confusing jargon. Some examples are:

Terms Synonymous with MBD	*Behavioral Disorders Attributed to MBD*
Association deficit pathology	Aggressive behavior disorder
Cerebral dysfunction	Aphasoid syndrome

Terms Synonymous with MBD	*Behavioral Disorders Attributed to MBD*
Cerebral dys-synchronization syndrome	Attention disorders
Diffuse brain damage	Character impulse disorder
Minimal brain damage	Conceptually handicapped
Minimal brain injury	Dyslexia
Minimal cerebral injury	Hyperexcitability syndrome
Minimal chronic brain syndromes	Hyperkinetic behavior syndrome
Minor brain damage	Hyperkinetic impulse disorder
Neurophrenia	Hyperkinetic syndrome
Organic behavior disorder	Hypokinetic syndrome
Organic brain damage	Interjacent child
Organic brain disease	Learning disabilities
Organic brain dysfunction	Perceptual cripple
Organic drivenness	Perceptually handicapped
	Primary reading retardation
	Psychoneurological learning disorders
	Specific reading disability

From Children's Learning and Attention Problems *by Kinsbourne and Caplan (Boston: Little, Brown and Company, 1979).*

In 1962, a multidisciplinary task force was formed to develop an acceptable definition of MBD, and in 1966 the following was published:

> Children of near average, average, or above average general intelligence with certain learning or behavioral disabilities ranging from mild to severe, which are associated with deviations of function of the central nervous system. These deviations may manifest themselves by various combinations of impairment in perception, conceptualization, language, memory, and control of attention, impulse, or motor function.

In 1968, the First Annual Report of the National Advisory Committee on Handicapped Children proposed the following definition (cited in Wiederhold, 1974):

> Children with special learning disabilities exhibit a disorder in one or more of the basic psychological processes involved in

> understanding or using spoken or written language. These may be manifested in disorders of listening, thinking, talking, reading, writing, spelling, or arithmetic. They include conditions which have been referred to as perceptual handicaps, brain injury, minimal brain dysfunction, dyslexia, developmental aphasia, etc. They do not include learning problems which are due primarily to visual, hearing, or motor handicaps, to mental retardation, emotional disturbance, or to environmental disadvantage.

The term *minimal* is unfortunate. It is used to differentiate this condition from the major brain disturbances in which there is obvious, gross pathology, such as cerebral palsy or major mental retardation, and in which pathology can often be seen with the naked eye and always on microscopic examination of the brain. On the contrary, the brains of children with MBD who have died from unrelated causes appear normal to gross and microscopic examination. This does not mean there is no pathology; it only means that neuroscientists have not yet discovered how or where to look. Current research continues to disclose interesting findings.

There is certainly nothing minimal in those individuals who are truly afflicted with handicaps that affect them severely throughout their lifetimes. Many children with severe dyslexia are not properly diagnosed until ages 12 to 14. By this time they often have serious emotional problems that arise from repeated school failures. Many hyperkinetic children have, in addition to their learning problems and inability to sit still, serious difficulties learning how to socialize, and are further damaged by negative feedback. They have experienced peer and adult rejection beginning at about three years of age, and their emotional developmental pattern is often adversely affected to a severe degree.

It is also unfortunate that the term *minimal* seems to be associated in the minds of many legislators with *minor* or *unimportant*. When they apportion funds, it is this category that is usually short-changed. Therefore, these children, who are the most amenable to good remediation, get the least. Many followup studies, beginning decades ago, have shown that it is this group of children that eventually accounts for most of the young jail population. Funds properly applied to help this type of childhood school failure could often produce a healthy, happy, educated, taxpaying, voting adult.

NONSTANDARD VS. ACCEPTABLE REMEDIATION METHODS

The chronic handicaps that adversely affect learning and acceptable behavior require such prolonged medical as well as educational intervention that parents are particularly vulnerable to the appeal of any method that offers a quick cure. The history of medicine is replete with such nostrums; there are more in existence today than ever before. It takes a combination of scientifically oriented doctors; well-controlled, double-blind studies; and, if medication is involved, the use of placebos to prove the effectiveness of any form of therapy. Such safeguards are just as important in the educational as in the medical treatment of children with learning disorders and other developmental disabilities.

Most pediatric neurologists, plus doctors who specialize in behavioral and learning problems of children, favor direct special education remediation methods. It is particularly important that educational demands are not so great as to add to the child's emotional problems. It is also stressed that the child experience success, that the teacher be well trained, and that the class size be optimal (usually smaller than most state legislatures require).

Remedial methods that are suspect in their effectiveness are those that are based on various vitamins, diets, perceptual training methods, hypoglycemia, patterning, and optical training methods. These "cures" are akin to many highly questionable and spurious medical treatments that have come and gone in past years. They are based on theories rejected by experts who judge them ineffective, but their proponents become quite defensive when challenged. Many testimonials and anecdotal case studies are offered as evidence, but objective researchers using the same techniques have failed to duplicate these claims of effectiveness.

On the other hand, parents need to have a role that they feel will, by their dedication, ameliorate their child's disability. They do not want to be told that acceptance is a major part of their role; they will resist this by grasping at every available alternative, and they will see in any change evidence that vindicates their faith, even though these changes occur more from elapsed time and parental attention than from the latest treatment regimen. Therefore, it is important to reassure parents that there is something that can be done and that their participation is necessary. This something is not "curing" the learning disability but rather using educating techniques that acknowledge the child's limitations and utilize and build on the potential present in every child. The parents need medical and educational experts to identify what their particular child has to work with and what techniques to apply to develop these functions to their utmost. Given specific activities, the parent can be helped to resist false hopes. Even so, the hope for a normal child will be latently waiting to spring alive.

Vitamins

There are still those who advocate treatment of learning disabilities with large doses of vitamins. Recognized medical authorities agree that this "orthomolecular" or "megavitamin" therapy has no benefit. It does have the definite potential danger of most large-dose vitamin regimes. Vitamins A, D, and E have well-known toxic effects. Even vitamin C, which some have advocated in large doses for the common cold, can cause kidney stones.

Minerals

Copper and zinc are two of the various minerals that have been recommended as treatments for learning disability. As with vitamins, minerals provide no proven beneficial effect despite claims to the contrary. Also, toxic side effects are well documented.

Diets

The Feingold diet is now enjoying what will probably be a brief period of popularity as treatment for hyperactive children.

Its theoretical basis is that many foods and food dyes contain salicylates that cause hyperactivity in certain susceptible children.

Some of the earlier studies by other authorities were tentatively confirmatory, but all later work has failed to bear out the early optimism. It can now be stated that the diet is generally not helpful. The most that can be said is that it may be helpful in a small subset of hyperactive children. Besides, it is extremely difficult to prepare. The entire family must eat it if the child is expected to stay with it, and the child who already has a problem with peer relations is segregated even further during parties and snack times.

Hypoglycemia

Low blood sugar has been cited as a cause of learning disability. Though this is also unsubstantiated, hypoglycemia has become a "wastebasket" type of diagnosis for many common complaints of a vague behavioral or neurologic nature.

All physicians of considerable experience have seen patients with true hypoglycemia. It is both rare and serious. It must be very carefully diagnosed, usually under hospital conditions, and just as carefully treated. It is not to be considered as a cause of learning disability.

Allergy

Certain allergists state that some learning disorders are caused by allergies of the brain to certain specific foods or other substances. They have advocated allergic testing and desensitization treatments. They describe what has been called the *tension–fatigue* syndrome as a type of learning disability.

Again, none of this has been confirmed and is regarded as highly suspect by most medical experts.

Patterning

The patterning method, originating some 20 years ago as treatment for mental retardation, cerebral palsy, learning disability, and a host of other disorders, is also known as the Doman–Delacato method. It enjoyed wide popularity for many years and is now rarely used. Objective medical investigation has proved this treatment of no benefit, and it is even considered fraudulent by some. It is usually recommended for years, and treatment is very expensive. The false hopes given to the family delay the acceptance of the child's true condition and the initiation of realistic remedial educational methods.

Visual Training

Unfortunately, war has been declared along professional lines regarding the benefits of visual training in children with normal eyes to remediate learning disabilities. Many optometrists are sincerely dedicated to such treatment while ophthalmologists and neurologists regard it as useless.

In brief, the two sides of this controversy present the following arguments:

Optometry	Ophthalmology
1. Children with reading problems are helped by glasses and/or eye exercises.	1. If a child can see well (no refractive error) without glasses, glasses will not benefit his or her reading ability.
2. *Seeing* involves use of eyes. *Vision* includes what the eyes see *plus* how the brain interprets this. Glasses can improve vision.	2. There is no difference between *seeing* and *vision*. A child without refractive error should not wear glasses. The eyes cannot be contributing to the reading problem.
3. Eye exercises will help a child read since tracking and certain other eye movements are an integral part of reading.	3. Exercises are beneficial only in certain children with abnormal eye muscles, such as in cross-eye. They do not improve reading ability.

Caught in the middle of all the controversies are the teachers and parents. How do they know whom to believe? It is hardly possible for them to study the literature in the field, so they have no basis for an informed decision. At the present state of our knowledge about learning disability, the best course to follow is one of healthy skepticism about any single approach, especially if it seems simplistic or is widely disputed.

The American Academy of Pediatrics and the American Association of Ophthalmology issued a joint statement expressing five major positions:

1. "Learning disability and dyslexia ... require a multi-disciplinary approach from medicine, education, and psychology in diagnosis and treatment. Eye care should never be instituted in isolation when a patient has a reading problem.
2. "...There is no peripheral eye defect which produces dyslexia and associated learning disabilities.
3. "No known scientific evidence supports claims for improving the academic abilities of learning-disabled or dyslexic children with treatment based soley on:
   a. visual training (muscle exercise, ocular pursuit, glasses)
   b. neurologic organization (laterality training, balance board, perceptual training)
4. "Excluding correctable refractive errors such as myopia, hyperopia, and astigmatism, glasses have no value in the specific treatment of dyslexia or other learning problems.
5. "The teaching of learning-disabled and dyslexic children is a problem of educational science."

Most optometrists do a limited assessment, focusing on visual and visual motor areas of functioning but not on auditory and language areas. Thus, even if an optometric evaluation should indicate a certain type of visual disability, it will not necessarily rule out the possibility of the child having other areas of disability. A full special educational evaluation should cover all areas of possible disability. It should also integrate the therapy into the full learning process (like remedial reading or math) to assist the child's performance within the classroom.

Alpha Wave Conditioning

At one time biofeedback techniques were used experimentally for the alleviation of learning disability. Children suspected of having poorly organized alpha waves on an electroencephalogram were taught through feedback to control their alpha waves, and this was supposed to cure or help their learning disability. This, too, has been generally discarded.

Sensory Integrative Therapy

Sensory integrative therapy was advocated by A. J. Ayres and is rarely encountered today. It was assumed that maximum sensory stimulation would improve classroom performance. Examples of such exercises were: involving the sense of balance by postural changes such as spinning or skating; tactile stimulation like working puzzles; tactile stimulation from vibrating brushes, etc.

Perceptual–Motor Exercises

It has been noted that children with learning disabilities are often clumsy. For this and other reasons, various researchers have developed physical exercises that are designed to aid the child's perception of his or her body parts—self-image in the anatomical sense. Remedial procedures include walking on a narrow board, using a balancing board, trampoline exercises, rhythm exercises, and so on. Kephart has developed a theory that postulates a number of states through which a child must progress to regain all lost ground. This approach is somewhat similar to the Doman-–Delacato method, at least in theory, and its effectiveness is unproved. The children, however, love it. Its greatest value lies in getting the reading-disabled child out of the classroom and into an area of the school where he or she cannot only have fun but also succeed. The perceptual–motor exercises, if judiciously used, can be done in the school itself, thereby simultaneously combined with and related to a remedial reading program. The major benefit in a program of positive experience of this type is likely the result of enhancement of the child's self-concept, so it also helps if the child feels that the reason for doing the exercises is to help him or her learn to read. It is just as important for the remedial reading program to be carefully structured so the child succeeds at this task as well, no matter how simple it is.

Summary

There is evidence that indicates that approaches to reading that rely solely on visual, auditory, or kinesthetic training, but do not include some actual reading experience, may lead to negative attitudes toward reading in general. Therefore, it is important to steer an even course between nonreading approaches and academic approaches.

The best lesson to be learned from the foregoing material is that more and more ingenious remediation methods will undoubtedly be developed in the future. Educators as well as school nurses and physicians will need to exercise vigilance in their judgment. They will do well to join in a dialogue that pools their areas of expertise.

ROLE OF THE SCHOOL NURSE

Some of the suggested activities go beyond the traditional role of most school nurses. However, the activities suggested here are all performed by currently practicing school nurses and have been found to be helpful to both physician and school:

1. Monitor and, if possible, administer prescribed medication.
2. Interpret the medical aspects of the learning and/or behavior problem to educational personnel.
3. Observe classroom behavior. Is there evidence of hyperactivity, aggressive hostility, excessive withdrawal, or other unusual behaviors? See the Connors Checklist. It can be reproduced and offered to the classroom teacher. Its

advantage is its brevity and the fact that it has been standardized. It should be filled out by the classroom teacher and an impartial observer such as the school nurse. It can then be given to the parent to show to the physician or, with parental permission, sent directly to the physician.

4. Maintain telephone contact with the physician. Physicians usually get their feedback only from the parents. An informed school nurse can furnish accurate medical or nursing information from the school as well. This dual reporting will help the child's physician serve the patient more effectively.
5. Conduct parent conferences at school and at home. Children with learning disabilities are usually bright in most cognitive areas, and, if the consultation process is unduly prolonged, it doesn't take children very long to receive the message that the parents cannot accept them as they are. This merely reaffirms their already held belief that they are not worth much, and makes the remediation efforts more difficult. Therefore, parents must guard against continual consultations with too many experts.
6. When appropriate, assist in development of the individual educational plan.
7. Develop and use other appropriate behavioral checklist forms to record student behavior objectively. See the example on page 204.

ABBREVIATED BEHAVIOR CHECKLIST

To be filled out by classroom teacher	0 Not at all	1 Just a little	2 Pretty much	3 Very much
1. Restless or overactive, excitable, impulsive				
2. Disturbs other children				
3. Fails to finish things started				
4. Short attention span				
5. Constant fidgeting				
6. Inattentive, easily distracted				
7. Demands must be met immediately				
8. Cries often and easily				
9. Mood changes quickly and drastically				
10. Temper outbursts, explosive and unpredictable behavior				

A check in any column is given as many points as indicated at the top of the column. A total of more than 15 to 20 points is said to confirm the diagnosis of hyperactivity.

SECTION 16

EMERGENCIES SEEN IN THE SCHOOL CLINIC

This section covers the nature and treatment of the many different kinds of emergencies that are seen in the school clinic, including:

- Lacerations of the skin
- Puncture wounds of the skin
- Fainting
- Injuries and foreign materials in eye, ear, nose
- Blood in anterior chamber (hyphema) of eye
- Arm and leg injuries
- Nosebleed
- Menstrual problems
- Bruise
- Muscle and joint pains
- Stomach ache
- Appendicitis
- Headache
- Vomiting
- Diarrhea
- Food poisoning
- Burns
- Injury to internal organs
- Head injuries
- Intracranial hemorrhage

It also provides information and guidelines regarding temperature measurement, including types of thermometers, normal temperature, fever, methods of measurement, and time of measurement.

LACERATIONS OF THE SKIN

Nature of the Condition

Emergency treatment and later management depend entirely on the nature of the laceration, which may be clean and straight or dirty and jagged. Because of a greater blood supply, lacerations of the face and scalp usually bleed more profusely than those on other body parts. This greater blood supply, however, leads to better healing.

Treatment and School Relevance

Pain

Most lacerations seen at school are not very severe and rarely require medication to control pain. If the pain is severe, a physician must be consulted.

Bleeding

The best way to control bleeding is to place a gauze flat directly on the cut and press firmly with a finger or the palm of the hand. (See Figure 16–1.) After three to five minutes of pressure, the bleeding will usually stop.

Pressure over pressure points is often advocated in some books on first aid. This does no harm but is rarely effective in slowing the blood flow.

Tourniquet application is controversial because, if applied too tightly and left on too long, the fingertips or toes may become gangrenous (die) from lack of blood supply. On the other hand, for severe bleeding a tight tourniquet is absolutely essential. What is safe? For severe bleeding, especially arterial bleeding in which blood is spurting, apply a tight tourniquet 1 or 2 inches above the wound, note the time, and never leave it on for more than 10 or 15

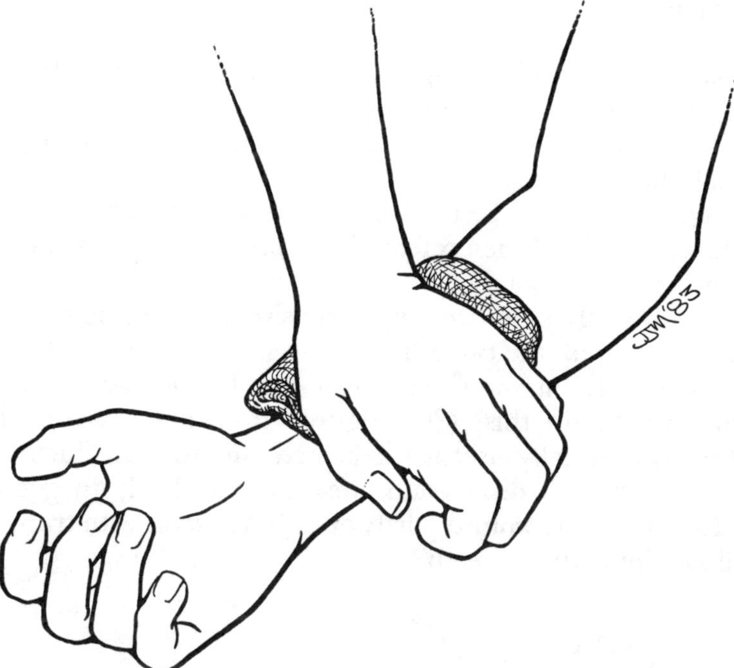

Figure 16–1. Applying pressure to large bleeding surface. (Amount of pressure should only be enough to stop bleeding—no more.)

minutes. The child must be immediately evacuated to an emergency medical facility.

Prevention of Infection

If the wound becomes infected, the resulting scar will be larger. Copious amounts of soap and water should be applied to wash out all dirt and other contaminating materials. This may be a bit painful at first, but it is highly necessary. The water should be lukewarm and may be running from a tap or in a soaking basin. Germicidal soap is all right but not necessary; plain soap is about as beneficial.

Merthiolate, mercurochrome, or other skin antiseptics may be used but not relied on to prevent infection. Iodine is quite painful and does no more good than any other skin antiseptic.

Dressing

Small cuts, after cleansing, may be covered with an adhesive bandage as the only treatment required. The bandage should be changed and the cut washed with soap and water daily till almost completely healed.

Larger cuts should be covered with a nonsticking gauze flat and adhesive tape and then referred to a physician right away, not at the end of the school day.

For a butterfly tape dressing, adhesive tape can be cut in a certain shape to pull the two edges of the skin together so that on healing the scar is narrower and sutures are not necessary. There are two ways to do this. (See Figures 16–2 and 16–3.) This procedure is especially useful for jagged cuts that are incurred under contaminated, dirty conditions and are likely to get infected. By leaving the wound partly open, an abscess with trapped pus will not form underneath.

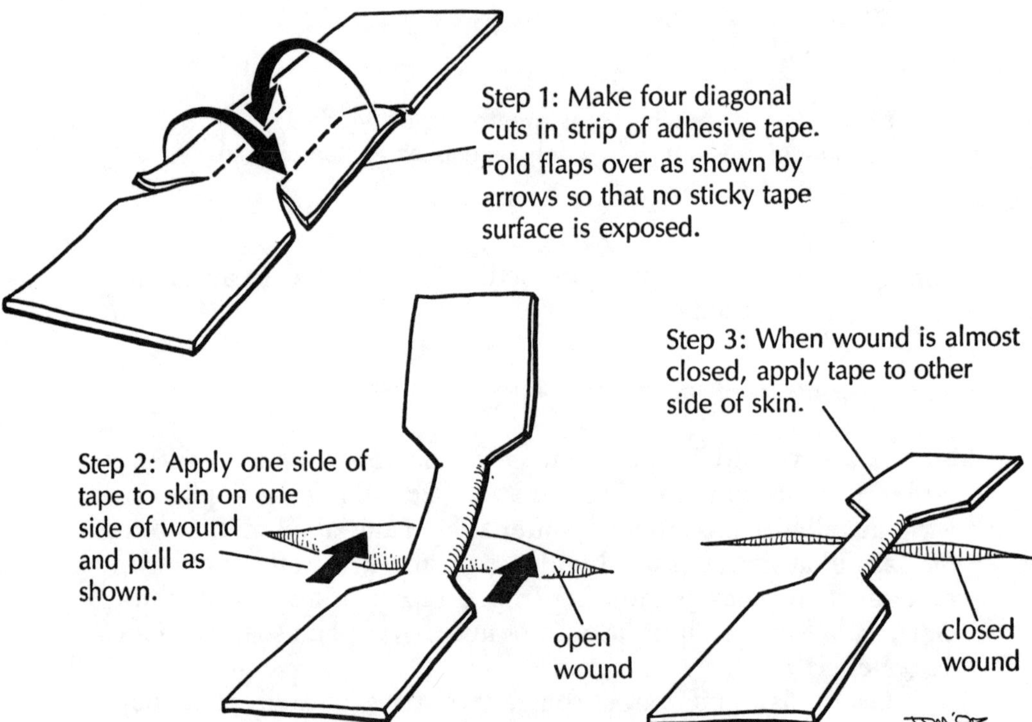

Figure 16–2. Adhesive tape strip butterfly dressing. (Size is usually about ¾ inch in width and ¾ inch in length.)

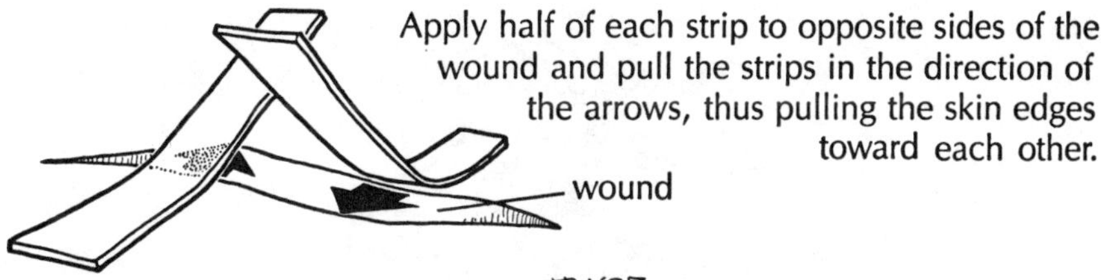

Figure 16–3. Alternative type of butterfly bandage. (Using two strips of adhesive tape about ¼ to ½ inch in width and 2 to 3 inches in length).

Sutures

Whether or not a cut will require stitches is a highly individual matter. Several factors must be considered.

1. Size and shape
   a. Jagged, irregular cuts or cuts longer than 1 inch, with the skin edges separated by ⅜ inch or greater usually need stitches.
   b. Cuts under ½ inch long with edges separated by ⅛ inch or less rarely need stitches.
2. Location
   a. Cuts on the face, especially the lip or eyelid, need careful attention regardless of size, sometimes by a plastic surgeon. (See Figures 16–4 and 16–5.)

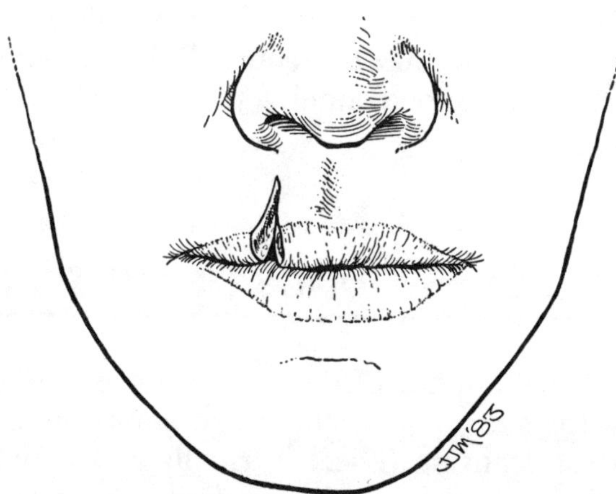

Figure 16–4. Laceration of upper lip

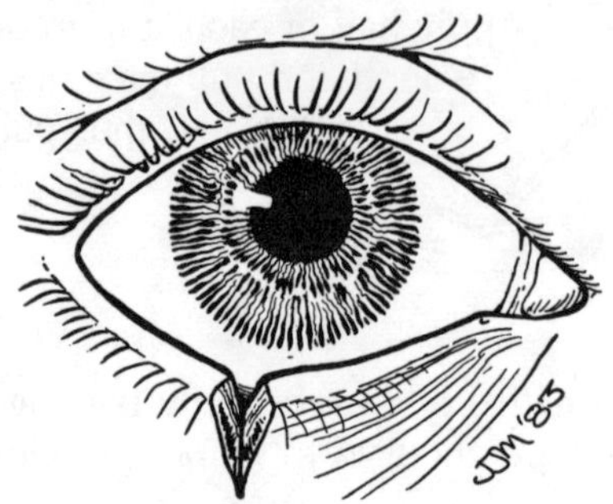

Figure 16–5. Laceration of lower eyelid

b. Cuts on the scalp should be seen by a physician. Hair tends to mat in the scab, delay healing, and occasionally, lead to infection.
c. Cuts inside the mouth, though the initial appearance may be bad, usually heal excellently with little or no scar.

3. Age—Only fresh cuts should be stitched (less than four to six hours). Older cuts should be taped loosely with the skin edges apart, so any infection will not be trapped under the skin edges and form an abscess (boil).

Booster Shots

If a child with a small clean cut has had a recent dose of tetanus toxoid, a booster shot will probably not be necessary. However, if the cut is large and dirty, or the child has not had a recent booster shot, one may be required. This decision should never be made by school personnel; a physician should always be consulted.

PUNCTURE WOUNDS OF THE SKIN

Most puncture wounds of the skin that are caused by small clean objects (pins or paper clips) are minor and need no treatment except cleansing. There is usually no bleeding, and an adhesive bandage should not be applied. (A dab of colored antiseptic may be applied so the child doesn't feel neglected.)

If a child steps on a nail or other sharp object, it is apt to be quite painful and the danger of infection is greater because any germs present will be deposited more deeply into the tissues. The foot should be soaked in warm water for 20 to 30 minutes. Epsom salts or another weak antiseptic may be used. This soaking encourages the wound to remain open and drain as much as possible.

After drying, a loose-fitting covering may be applied so air can enter. If the sole of the foot has been punctured, a small round pad with a hole in the center may be used to relieve pressure. Deciding whether or not to give a booster shot of tetanus toxoid requires the consideration of many factors. Nurses or other school personnel should not make the decision; a physician should be consulted.

A puncture wound with the point of a wooden pencil is often seen at school. Many individuals are often unduly concerned because they fear lead poisoning. The so-called lead in a pencil actually has no lead in it at all; it is compressed graphite, completely inert and nontoxic. It does color the skin and tissue immediately beneath and leaves a small bluish dot which is often permanent; it is actually a small tattoo.

Because of the bluish color, one gets the impression that the pencil tip is broken off under the skin. It is very rare that this happens. Unless one can see and feel the actual broken-off point of the pencil sticking up over the skin surface, efforts at removal usually result in greater tissue damage and should not be carried out. Treatment should be limited to cleansing to prevent infection as in any other small puncture wound. If the mark is on the face and is considered unsightly, it may be removed later by plastic surgery.

FAINTING

Nature of the Condition

Fainting can occur for a variety of reasons, such as weakness, hunger, strong emotional reactions, severe pain, or onset of an illness. Some individuals are more prone to faint than others. For unknown reasons, it is more common in girls.

Fainting usually is associated with a sudden decrease in blood supply to the brain and may or may not be associated with low blood pressure and slow pulse. Sudden change in position, especially from a lying or sitting to a standing position, can cause dizziness or even fainting.

Diagnosis and Symptoms

Fainting must be differentiated from an epileptic attack. In a simple fainting spell there are usually no twitching movements of the arms and legs. If there is any twitching, a physician will be required to rule out epilepsy. (See Section 7.)

Treatment and School Relevance

1. Place the head on the same level with or lower than the chest. If dizziness occurs while sitting in a chair, lower the head between the knees. A child who has fainted and is lying on the floor should remain there until recovery.
2. Check pulse and respiration. If they are normal, one can be reassured that the child will soon recover.
3. Blood pressure should be measured if possible. If the pressure is not excessively low (below 90/60), the fainting spell is less likely to be serious.
4. Many school nurses and teachers know which children in school are habitual fainters. When a child faints who has never fainted before, one must be much more cautious and suspect more serious causes.
5. Attempts to awaken the child do not help the child; they only reassure the nurse or teacher. It is better to observe the child for a short time and check the blood pressure, pulse, and respiration. If all signs point to deepening unconsciousness, then one should try to awaken the child. If the child moves or groans, it is an indication that he or she is not deeply unconscious; if not, emergency evacuation to a hospital or doctor's office is appropriate.

INJURIES AND FOREIGN MATERIALS

Eye

A speck of dirt, a cinder, or another tiny foreign object that suddenly lodges in the eye causes sudden pain and excessive tearing. Chemicals or other liquid irritants can cause lasting damage and need rapid special treatment. Cuts or bruises of the eye require special types of care.

1. If the child is cooperative and quiet, the lower lid can be pulled down and away from the eyeball. (See Figure 16–6.) This

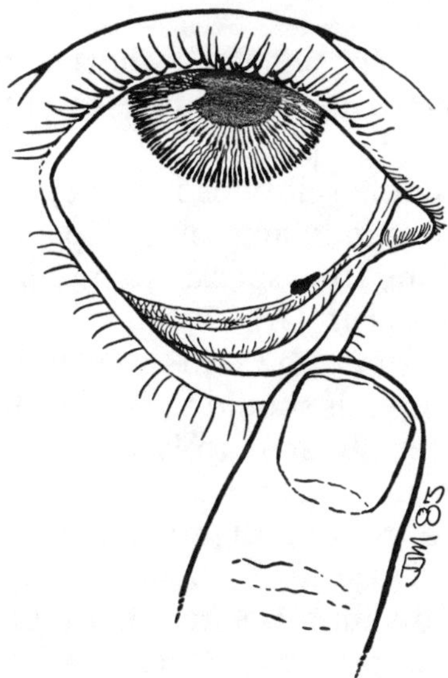

Figure 16–6. Foreign body in lower lid

may loosen the foreign body and allow the tears to wash it away. If the object is easy to see resting on the upper or lower lid (not on the eyeball), it can be safely removed with a cotton-tipped applicator. (See Figure 16–7.) In all other circumstances the child should be encouraged to blink frequently and not to rub the eye. If the foreign body is not gone after five to ten minutes, an eye

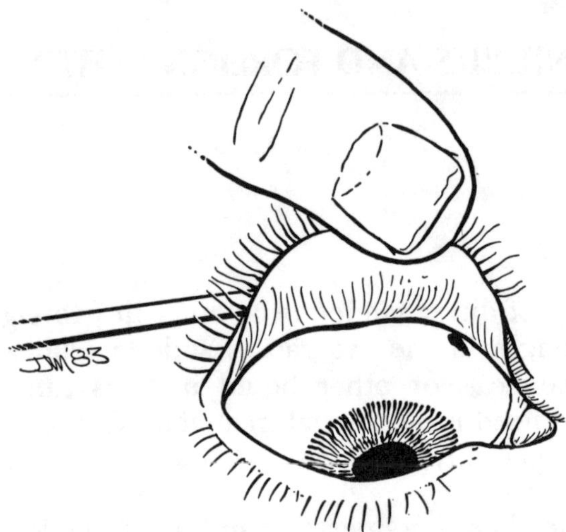

Figure 16–7. Foreign body in upper lid. (Lid is rolled back over a cotton swab.)

specialist should be consulted. If the child is sent to an eye specialist, the affected eye should be covered with a 2-inch by 2-inch gauze flat held in place with criss-crossed adhesive strips.

2. Acid or alkaline solutions in the eye must be washed out immediately with copious amounts of plain tap water. Do not waste time searching for special neutralizing solutions. It is important to use water in large volumes, not to squirt it into the eye in a small jet stream with rapid force. Ideally, the child should be lying down, the eyelids should be held wide open, and a gentle stream of cool water about ¼ to ½ inch in diameter should be allowed to run into the eye at the inner corner and out of the outer corner, so the head must be slightly tilted toward the side of the affected eye. (See Figure 16–8.) In any emergency of this nature, never be concerned with a wet bed, floor, or clothes. The above described physical apparatus is rarely available at a school. As a substitute, a team of three people can help calm the child and hold the lids open, slowly pour a glass of water into the inner corner of the eye, and keep another glass of water constantly filled so flushing is uninterrupted. Most acid and alkaline solutions are sticky; the water should run for 15 to 30 minutes. It is important to flush the eye first; then a 4-inch by 4-inch gauze flat should be taped over the eye, and the child should be taken directly to an eye specialist. A judgment must be made about how long to continue irrigation before taking the child to the eye doctor. If the

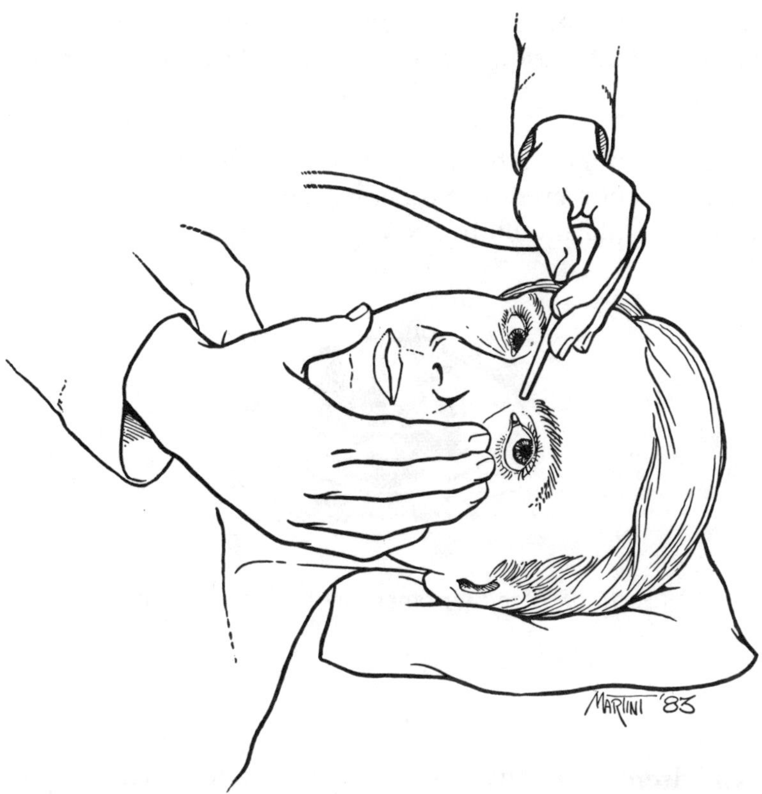

Figure 16–8. Flushing chemical irritant from eye. (Upper lid must be held up also.)

irrigation is proceeding smoothly and effectively, continue longer. If it seems ineffective and little water is actually flushing over the surface of the eyeball, go to the doctor sooner.

3. There are many ways for an eye to be injured by a blow, a cut, a penetrating injury, a burn, and so on. In all of these cases there will be an obvious need for quick referral to an eye specialist. The child will hold the hand over the eye, usually crying and complaining of pain or rubbing the eye excessively. In these obvious cases, a 4-inch by 4-inch gauze flat should be taped over the eye, and the child should be sent to the doctor immediately. *There is one type of eye injury that is serious but may escape detection by the school nurse or teacher unless it is suspected and looked for.* A blunt blow to the eyeball, such as with a baseball or a smooth round rock, may cause an injury to the cornea and anterior chamber (front part of the eyeball). The pain subsides after a relatively short time, but the cornea may be damaged and a small amount of blood may collect

in the anterior chamber. (See Figure 16–9.) If significant corneal injury is present, vision will be blurred. The only sure way to detect this is to test the child's visual acuity, preferably on the Snellen Test Chart. If the test chart is not available, the child should read letters in a book with one eye at a time. Vision should be equal in both eyes. If vision in the injured eye is poor or blurred, the child should be seen by an eye specialist immediately.

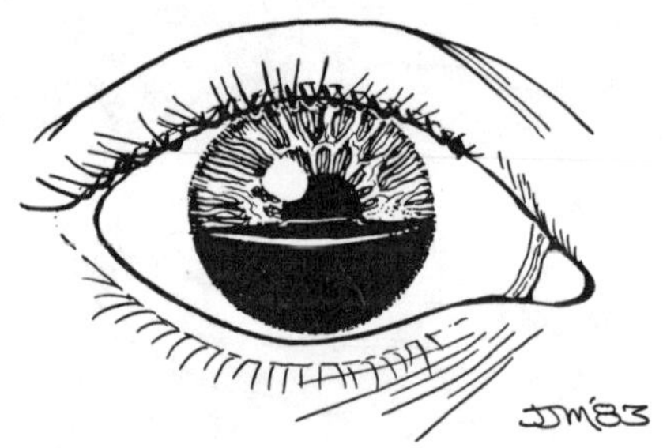

Figure 16–9. Blood (or other fluid) in anterior chamber.

Ear

Children often push erasers, paper wads, beans, or other objects into their ears. (See Figure 16–10.) This usually causes no pain, so the child usually doesn't report it. It is usually discovered during a later routine physical checkup.

Occasionally an insect will fly into the ear. Children will complain because of the buzzing and movement, not pain.

Nurses or other school personnel should never try to remove any foreign object from the ear unless it is sticking out and can be easily grasped with the fingers or forceps. Foreign objects in the ear are quite difficult to get out. Without the proper equipment, special technique, and good lighting, the object will be pushed in further.

If an insect is in the ear, it is safe to kill it with alcohol; never use mineral oil because it may cause the insect to swell up and make later removal more difficult.

Foreign bodies in the ear are not emergency conditions but should be referred to a physician as soon as feasible.

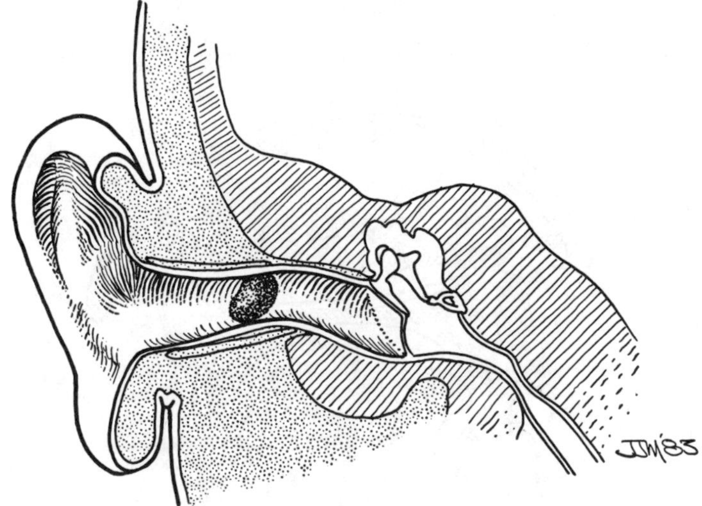

Figure 16–10. Foreign body in ear.

Nose

Children push the same objects into their noses as they do into their ears. (See Figure 16–11.) There is no pain, and parents or school personnel are never told. However, since the nose is always moist, infection ensues and causes nasal discharge from only one nostril, with a foul odor. Nasal discharge from a common cold, sinus, or allergy is seen on both sides and rarely is associated with a foul odor.

Exactly the same warnings apply as for foreign bodies in the ear. Occasionally a child will report a foreign body in the nose. Unless it is sticking out, any attempts to remove it will just push it in further.

This is not an emergency condition, but the child should be referred to a physician as soon as feasible.

Trauma to the nose must be treated with caution; a fracture may cause later disfigurement. If there is any doubt, the child should be seen by a physician for x-rays.

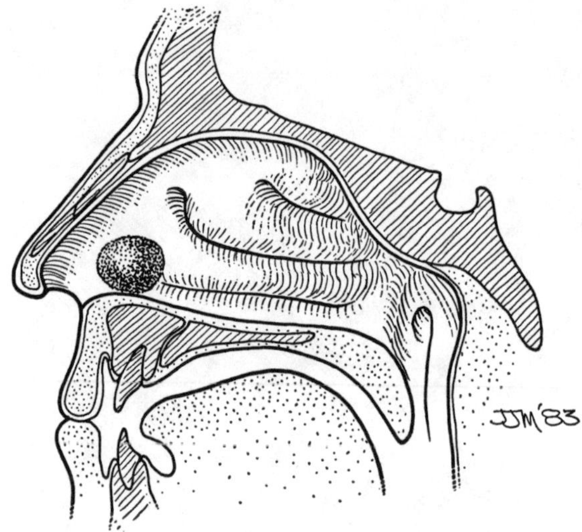

Figure 16–11. Foreign body in nose.

ARM AND LEG INJURIES

Sprain and Strain

Nature of the Condition

A *sprain* is a stretching injury of a ligament that does not actually tear it. A *strain* is a stretching injury of a muscle or tendon that does not actually cause the tendon or muscle to tear or rupture. (See Figure 16–12.)

Either of these injuries can be mild or severe, requiring only a little rest in mild cases or an actual plaster cast in severe cases. They usually occur during athletic contests in secondary school but may also occur during normal childhood play, especially during recess.

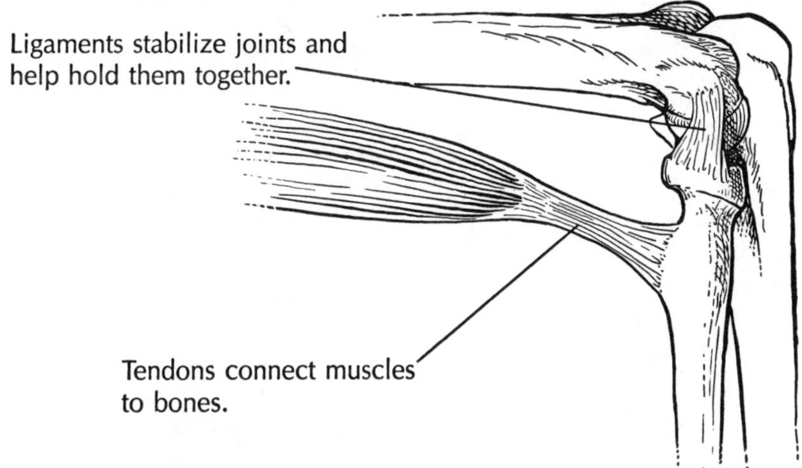

Figure 16–12. Difference between tendon and ligament.

Symptoms

There is pain and swelling, of sudden onset, after twisting the ankle, knee, wrist, elbow, shoulder, hand, or foot.

Treatment

ICE stands for ice, compression, and elevation. Ice can be safely applied directly to the skin, but it is much more comfortable if the ice is first wrapped in a towel. Compression should never be performed by untrained personnel—cutting off the blood supply presents a serious danger. Elevation is often helpful.

Refer to a physician in all but very mild cases.

Fractures

Nature of the Condition

A fractured bone is a broken bone; there is no difference. There are numerous different kinds of fractures, but most have

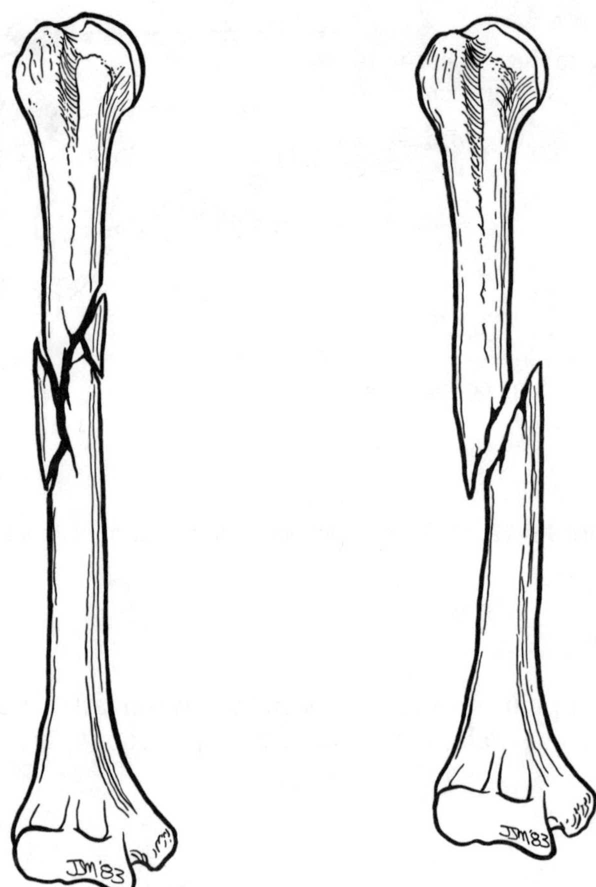

Figure 16–13. Comminuted fracture. **Figure 16–14.** Oblique fracture.

one thing in common—they will not heal properly unless put in some type of cast. (See Figures 16–13 through 16–18.)

Symptoms

Pain and swelling and sometimes crookedness can be seen in the fractured arm or leg. In many minor fractures the bones are not out of line, but special treatment such as a cast is necessary for proper healing.

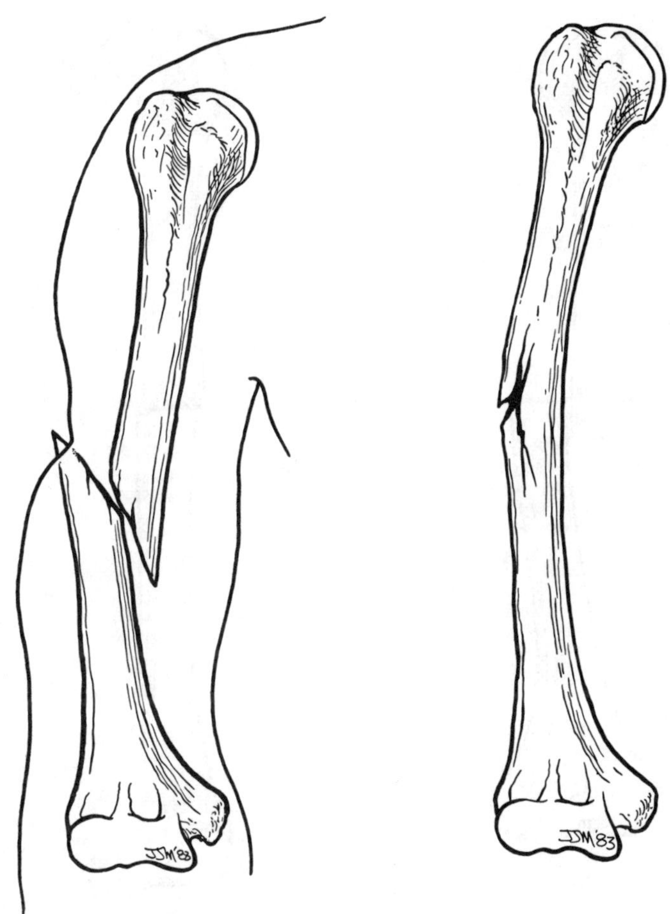

Figure 16–15. Compound fracture. **Figure 16–16.** Greenstick fracture.

During the healing process new bone is built up around the fracture site; this new bone is called *callus.* It often causes a knot or bump that goes away after complete healing.

Treatment and Diagnosis

Any suspected fracture should always be referred to a physician. The diagnosis can only be made with certainty by x-ray. The treatment is by splint and sling.

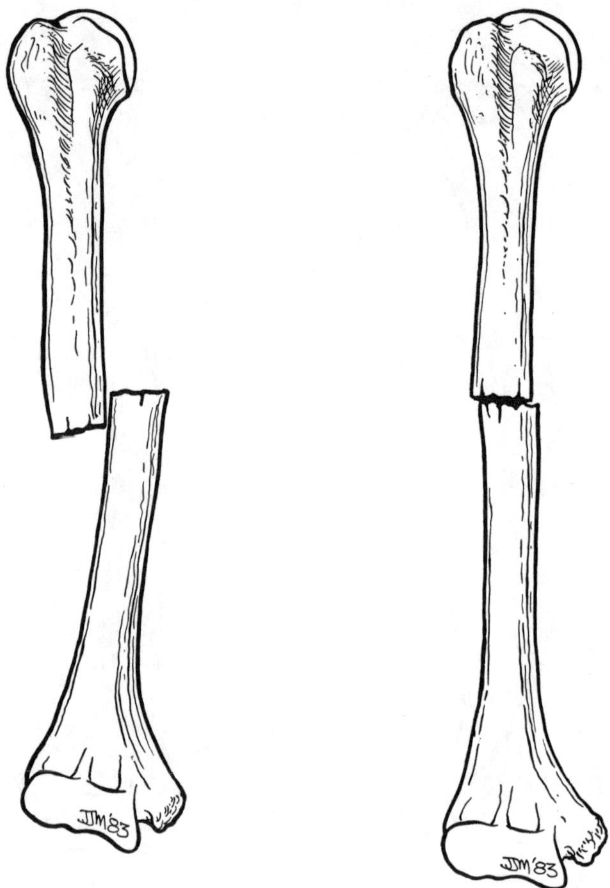

Figure 16–17. Displaced fracture. **Figure 16–18.** Nondisplaced fracture.

Dislocations

Nature of the Condition

In school-age children dislocation is most apt to occur in the ball-and-socket joint of the shoulder. (See Figure 16–19.) This may occur following an injury or from throwing a ball too hard. If the elbow, wrist, ankle, knee, or hip becomes dislocated, it usually follows a severe injury and is often accompanied by a fracture.

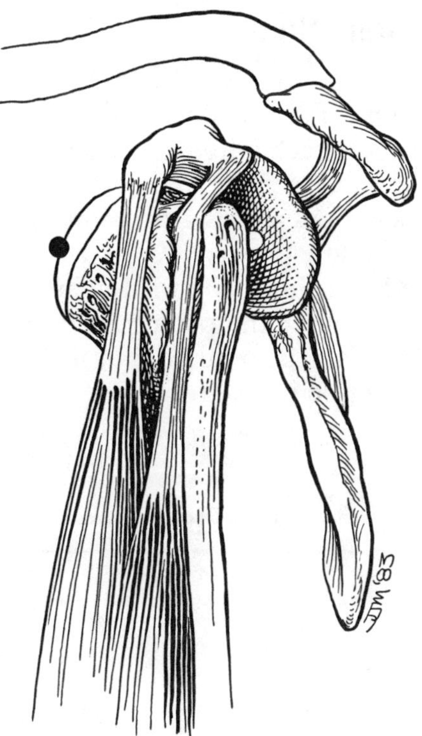

Figure 16–19. Rotation-type dislocation of shoulder. (The shoulder is a ball-and-socket joint. The ball is the upper end of the humerus. The ball's apex is shown by the black dot. The socket is at the lateral plate of the scapula or shoulder blade. When the dislocation is reduced, back in place, the black dot will fit into the white hole.)

Symptoms

Severe pain and noticeable deformity are always present.

Treatment

After ice application the child should always be referred to a physician, preferably an orthopedic surgeon. *Definitive treatment (putting the joint back in place) should never be attempted at school.* This may look easy in the case of a dislocated finger joint, but school nurses, coaches, and athletic trainers should resist the temptation.

Role of the School Nurse

Sprains, strains, fractures, and dislocations are common occurrences at school. Each school should develop a prearranged plan with contacts made in advance at a doctor's office or a hospital emergency room so hasty decisions need not be made in an acute emergency situation.

These procedures should be written and, if possible, posted in the nurse's clinic and/or the principal's office.

Parents must always be notified, but if they are not available, treatment should not be delayed.

NOSEBLEED

Nature of the Condition

Though nosebleeds are very common in elementary-school-age children, they are rarely serious. They occur more frequently in boys during hot weather. Repeated nosebleeds are often viewed with alarm, but unless one sees bleeding in other areas of the body (blood spots under the skin, bleeding in the urine, etc.), or unless the nosebleed cannot be stopped with simple measures, it is rare that a medical referral is necessary, unless the bleeding follows a blow to another part of the head.

Nosebleeds are more common in any child with irritation of the nose such as occurs in allergy or colds. Also, such children are apt to pick their noses and thus break tiny blood vessels. Therefore, repeated nosebleeds in the same child are quite common.

Treatment

A key or ice pack on the back of the neck is ineffective.

A slightly effective method is pressing on the upper lip

against the teeth or placing a long flat object between the teeth and upper lip.

Most effective is pressing the ends of the nose together quite firmly between thumb and forefingers for five minutes (by the clock). Have the child breathe through the open mouth.

In almost all nosebleeds the ruptured blood vessel is near the tip end of the nose, and direct pressure is always the best way to stop any bleeding. If one can see that only one side is bleeding, pressure is necessary on that side only.

The child should be in a sitting position with the upper body leaning forward. The forehead may be rested on a wall or shelf, if desired.

After the bleeding stops, the child should remain in the school clinic for 15 to 20 minutes. If bleeding does not recur, the child may go back to class.

Role of the School Nurse

The child should be excused from recess or other outdoor physical activity for that day only. Parents should be notified. Medical referral is necessary only in severe nosebleeds (more than 15 to 30 minutes), frequently recurring nosebleeds, or bleeding in other body areas.

MENSTRUAL PROBLEMS

Nature of the Condition

The medical problems associated with menstruation fall under the following three categories:

1. Pain
2. Excessive bleeding
3. Unexpected bleeding

Symptoms

Excessive menstrual pain—*dysmenorrhea*—is very common in school-age girls. It usually begins one to three years after the *menarche* (onset of menstruation) and practically always disappears after the birth of the first child. The pain can be very severe and accompanied by vomiting, headache, and backache. In severe cases, a day or two of school may be missed each month.

Excessive bleeding means either more frequent than approximately once a month, or once a month but excessive in amount.

Normal menstruation does not occur more often than 21 days from the first day of one period to the first day of the next, the bleeding does not last more than 6 days, and not more than six well-soaked pads are used every 24 hours.

Unexpected bleeding can be caused by unexpected menarche or unexpected onset of a period in a previously menstruating girl.

Treatment and School Relevance

For pain:

1. Have the girl lie down in school clinic.
2. Give aspirin or Tylenol.
3. Send the patient home if pain is severe.
4. Refer her to a physician if pain continues.

There are several medications that are very helpful in preventing dysmenorrhea. They must be prescribed by a physician and are quite safe.

For excessive bleeding:

1. More frequent than about once a month—refer to a physician; nothing can be done at school.
2. Excessive bleeding during regular period—refer to a physician.

For unexpected bleeding:

1. Unexpected onset of menarche—supply with sanitary napkins, allow to rest in clinic, provide emotional support

and brief pertinent educational information to relieve fears.
2. Unexpected onset of period in a previously regular girl—refer to a physician.

Role of the School Nurse

1. Provide a quiet, private place for the girl to rest.
2. Administer aspirin or Tylenol with parents' and physician's permission.
3. Provide reassurance and menstrual information.
4. Suggest that the student keep a calendar so onset of menstruation will not be unexpected.

BRUISE

Nature of the Condition

A bruise occurs following sudden impact from a fall or blow by a rock, fist, or other blunt object. The surface of the skin is not broken, but the underlying blood vessels are ruptured and the surrounding tissues are crushed and damaged. In medical jargon, it is called a *contusion.*

Symptoms

Pain, redness, and swelling will usually be seen. If the bruise is minor, no redness or swelling will result. At first the blood in the tissues causes reddish discoloration. In a few days the blood gets older and turns bluish-purple and then yellowish-green. This color change demonstrates the age of the bruise. Swelling usually disappears within four days, depending on the severity of the bruise and its location. Pain lasts a few minutes in minor bruises, but tenderness persists for days in more severe bruises.

Diagnosis

This is usually obvious from the history and symptoms. However, a child with a disease that causes a delay in blood clotting may be seen with an identical-looking condition and no history of pain or trauma. If the history is reliable, one should examine the child to see if any other bruises are present. If there are, the child should be sent home at the end of the day with a note to the parent.

Treatment

An ice pack will relieve pain. If no ice is readily available, a towel wrung out with cold tap water will help. Commercially available products that produce instant cold packs are available. It would be well to store some of these at each school.

Compression bandages, when indicated, should never be applied by untrained personnel. The danger of cutting off the blood supply is too great. If the injury looks severe, the child should be sent home or to a hospital emergency room with a loose-fitting cold pack.

Elevation of an injured arm with a sling or propping a leg on a chair is helpful.

The procedure outlined above is commonly referred to as ICE treatment, an acronym for ice, compression, and elevation. The same treatment is effective for joint injuries such as sprained ankle or twisted knee, shoulder, or elbow.

Role of the School Nurse

Assess the severity of the bruise. If it is minor yet needs treatment, it may be treated at school; if it is severe, the child should be sent home or to a medical facility.

Be on the alert for nontraumatic discolorations of the skin that resemble bruises; this sometimes occurs spontaneously and is often completely painless. If they are on the body or arms, they may have more serious import and, if more than one is seen, parents should be notified. A blood clotting disease may be present.

Warning: Children often have several bruises on their legs, especially between the ankle and knee, and have no knowledge of any injury. These occur during the rough-and-tumble of normal childhood play and need no treatment at all. Also, some adolescent girls (and older women) bruise very easily, such as from a slight bump on the corner of a desk. Bruises limited to the thighs and legs in these individuals need no treatment.

Bruises are one of the most common occurrences a school nurse is called upon to treat. Most children need only a little reassurance, some need ice for relief of pain, and very few need to be seen by a physician.

Be aware that bruises in different stages of healing on various parts of the body may be warning signals of child abuse.

MUSCLE AND JOINT PAINS NOT INJURY-RELATED

Nature of the Condition

Pain in the arms and legs occurs in children who have not been injured, much more often in the legs than in the arms, so pain in the arms must be taken more seriously. The pain may be in the muscles or in the joints; the significance and treatment are quite different.

Neck pain (crick in the neck), commonly seen at school, can result from several factors such as sound sleep with the neck in a stressed or twisted position, or excessive cold causing neck muscle tension. Arthritis of a cervical (neck) bone, very rare in children, may simulate a crick.

Nontraumatic muscle pain is almost always caused by excessive use during normal childhood play. This is from excessive lactic acid production, a byproduct of muscle glycogen metabolism that causes delayed pain by irritation of the muscle. This goes away quickly without intervention. A related condition, growing pains, occurs for the same reason, always in the legs, and it characteristically awakens a child from sleep.

Nontraumatic joint pain may indicate some type of arthritis. It is rare and should be regarded cautiously if it occurs.

Symptoms

Pain is the usual symptom, though redness and swelling may be seen in certain types of arthritis. It is quite common for the pain to occur an hour or two following a play period.

Diagnosis

Differentiation between muscle pain and joint pain is very important; the treatment is different. The best way to tell the difference is by gentle manipulation. Any movement or massage of a diseased joint will usually cause increased pain; gentle massage to a painful, noninjured muscle usually brings relief.

Treatment

Cold applications, by numbing nerve endings and slowing blood circulation, diminish pain and swelling.

Heat applications, by increasing blood circulation, increase tissue metabolism and thus promote healing and return to a normal condition.

Therefore, most traumatic pains are treated with cold, whereas nontraumatic muscle and joint pains are best treated with heat. A heat lamp can provide excellent relief in some cases, but care must be taken not to burn the skin. Hot wet compresses are equally effective.

Gentle massage can sometimes provide relief, especially if the pain is in the calf muscles. If any manipulation increases the pain, it must be stopped immediately.

Athletes are often advised to exercise a painful muscle to work out the pain. This method should not be used in younger children. At best *it should only be used after the cause of the pain is carefully diagnosed by a trained professional.*

Role of the School Nurse

If the pain is minor and of short duration, the student can be sent back to class.

If manipulation causes increased pain, stop treatment and allow the child to rest in the clinic. If pain goes away, send the child back to class. If pain persists an hour or more, send the child home.

Emergency evacuation is not necessary unless pain is very severe.

STOMACH ACHE

Nature of the Condition

All children have stomach aches occasionally. The causes are numerous. It is by far the most common childhood complaint, and most of the time the condition is minor, needs no special treatment, and goes away by itself. Stomach aches can also be caused by emotional distress. This does not mean the child is emotionally disturbed; it is simply his or her particular reaction to stress. Other children may react to stress with a headache. One of the most common causes of stomach aches is *mesenteric adenitis.* This means swelling of the lymph nodes in the abdomen, a temporary condition that may accompany many common childhood diseases, such as the common cold, influenza, or chicken pox.

Emotional causes of stomach ache are extremely varied. Some of the more common are:

1. School academic failure
2. Not liking the teacher (or vice versa)
3. Being harassed by a bully on the playground or around school
4. Parental or sibling anxiety, child abuse, or other home problems
5. School phobia

Though some older children can talk about problems of this nature, it is usually unrealistic to expect it of younger children.

Symptoms and Treatment

1. *Fever.* This can only be determined by using a thermometer and indicates an organic cause (as opposed to emotional). It is usually an indication for sending the child home. A child with a stomach ache without fever could possibly have something serious, but it is much less likely.

2. *Facial expression.* A child who complains of a stomach ache, looks alert, does not seem worried, or does not frown as if in pain, usually does not have a serious condition. Such a child needs to rest in the school clinic for a while, and if no fever is present and the pain is gone in ten or fifteen minutes, it is safe to send him or her back to class. Suggest that the child come back later if his or her stomach starts to hurt again.

3. *Vomiting or diarrhea.* If either of these symptoms is present, the child usually has a disease that is contagious, and he or she should be sent home.

4. *Position of comfort.* If the child is just as comfortable sitting in a chair as lying on a cot, it usually indicates a less serious type of stomach ache.

5. *Progression of pain.* In the more serious stomach aches, the pain usually gets worse after an hour or two; in the less serious, the pain usually diminishes within the first hour after onset.

APPENDICITIS

When a child with a stomach ache comes to the clinic, school personnel are concerned because *appendicitis,* if left untreated, can progress rapidly and lead to rupture with peritonitis (infection of the entire abdominal cavity), an extremely serious disease. While no school nurse or other school person should take the responsibility for making such a diagnosis, there are certain symptoms that should make one suspicious.

1. *Fever.* Early in the course of appendicitis the fever is low, 99.6 to 101 degrees Fahrenheit in most cases. For this reason it is most important to use a thermometer. It is impossible to detect a fever of 100 degrees by feeling a child's forehead.

2. *Location and progression of pain.* The pain characteristically begins in the pit of the stomach—in the center and just below the ribs—and as it increases in severity, it gradually moves to the lower right, halfway between the navel and the groin. The pain slowly but surely gets worse. This is an important symptom, characteristic of appendicitis. The speed of progression varies a great deal—the younger the child, the faster. In general, however, in a first to fifth grade child (ages six to eleven), the pain that begins in the pit of the stomach will have moved down to the lower right quadrant of the abdomen within two to six hours. In a three-year-old, progress is often faster.

3. *Facial expression.* The child with appendicitis does not come into the clinic smiling; he or she usually looks uncomfortable.

4. *Position of comfort.* In appendicitis, the child would rather lie down than sit up, often on the left side with the right leg drawn up.

5. *Other findings.* These include constipation, loss of appetite, and abdominal tenderness to pressure, but these symptoms are best evaluated by a physician. If appendicitis is suspected, the parents should be called and the child should be taken to the doctor immediately.

HEADACHE

Nature of the Condition

Headache is a common symptom of emotional anxiety as well as organic disease. One must assess many of the same factors seen in children with stomach aches. Fever and facial expression have the same import. A happy child without a fever does not in all likehood have a serious headache.

Some physicians feel that a child who misses breakfast may get a headache from hunger. Others do not agree. In any case, it never hurts to offer a child with a headache something to eat—if the child is hungry. Juice, milk, biscuits, or cookies in small amounts will do no harm. If the child is not hungry, it is better not to eat because it may precipitate vomiting.

The following accompanying symptoms are important warning signs and, if present, the child should be sent home:

1. Dizziness
2. Blurred vision
3. Fainting
4. Fever
5. Drowsiness
6. Vomiting
7. Persistence for an hour or more

Treatment and School Relevance

A short rest in the clinic is usually all that is necessary. However, many children have minor headaches fairly often, and parents will ask the school nurse or principal to give the child an aspirin whenever he or she complains of a headache. Parents, and sometimes even school personnel, are often unaware that all nurses, including school nurses, are prohibited by law from giving any medication—prescription or nonprescription—that is not ordered by a licensed physician. School nurses often fear action by their state licensing agency (loss of license) as well as later litigation by parents. Parents, on the other hand, simply cannot understand why a school nurse cannot do such a simple thing as give a child an aspirin or other nonprescription medication for an occasional headache. An easy solution to this dilemma is simply to ask the parent to bring a note from the physician authorizing the school nurse (or other delegated personnel) to administer the medicine. When this note is also signed by the parent, the school authorities will have sufficient legal protection.

VOMITING

Nature of the Condition

Nausea and vomiting are very common childhood complaints. Almost any illness can cause a child to vomit. At school the nurse must decide whether this symptom is the result of a disease for which the parent must be called and the child sent home, or whether simply to have the child lie down in the clinic for 10 to 20 minutes.

Causes

1. *Minor childhood illnesses*—There are literally hundreds of bacteria and viruses that cause gastrointestinal upsets in children, often associated with fever.
2. *Emotional anxiety.*
3. *Food poisoning*—Though this is often of primary concern in a school that serves meals, it is actually a rare occurrence. However, many children vomiting at about the same time should raise the suspicion that they ate spoiled or contaminated food from the school cafeteria.

Symptoms and Role of the School Nurse

One episode of vomiting does not necessarily mean the child needs to go to the doctor—or even go home from school. Vomiting one time only can be caused by too much exercise in the hot sun, strong emotional factors (fear, anxiety, etc.), or other factors that are not serious enough to send the child home.

Fever, as measured by the thermometer, is probably the most important factor to consider in assessment. When present, send the child home.

Facial expression, an important sign, should be assessed after a five- to ten-minute wait. If there is continued or increased discomfort, send the child home.

After the child vomits once, the school nurse should allow him or her to lie down in the clinic, take the temperature, and see how the child feels in 10 to 20 minutes. Then a decision should be made about whether to call the parents.

Blood in the vomitus is not necessarily a serious sign. On vomiting, the stomach muscles contract very tightly and frequently cause some of the smaller blood vessels to rupture. Therefore, many children who vomit, especially if they retch hard, will have some bloody streaks of mucus mixed with their stomach contents. The seriousness of the bleeding can be judged entirely by the amount of blood one sees. A few streaks should cause no alarm. Anything more than this, especially tablespoon quantities of blood, should be cause for emergency measures. Obviously, nothing can be done at school; arrangements should be made to transport the child to the nearest emergency room immediately, and then the parents should be notified immediately, in that order.

DIARRHEA

Nature of the Condition

Many of the same minor childhood diseases that cause vomiting can cause diarrhea in younger babies. However, school-age children who develop diarrhea usually have a specific intestinal disease. Many are caused by viruses, are minor, and are of short duration. Roughly half of the children with mild diarrhea have low-grade fever. This type of mild diarrhea usually lasts two or three days and goes away by itself.

Some children develop more severe diarrhea with higher

fever. These children are likely to have more stomach ache from intestinal cramping and will usually have most severe cramping pain just before another bowel movement. After the bowel movement the pain will diminish for a while. It is very rare for children with diarrhea to have only one loose stool and stop; they usually have more.

The contagiousness of any given case of diarrhea depends entirely on the cause. However, most cases are contagious, and appropriate precautions should be taken.

Symptoms and Role of the School Nurse

1. *Fever.* Children with mild diarrhea may have none at all; severe cases usually have more. When present, send the child home.
2. *Soiling of clothes at school.* This causes a child great distress. If facilities are available, the child should be cleaned up; if not, he or she should be helped home as quickly as possible.
3. *Stomach ache* (see page 221).
4. *Loss of appetite.*

Treatment

Kaopectate is one of the few medicines available that has no adverse side effects. It can be obtained over the counter and can be given in perfect safety according to directions on the bottle.

A child with diarrhea should not be urged to eat, but light foods in small quantities are all right if the child is hungry. To prevent dehydration and to maintain the flow of urine, liquids are important and should be urged.

Most cases are self-limiting and mild, especially in school-age children, and do not need to be seen by a doctor. However, severe cases with fever and cramps should be referred to a physician.

FOOD POISONING

Diagnosis

Fever is rarely present, though it may occur.

Check with the school medical consultant to see if there is an epidemic of gastrointestinal disease in the community or at other schools. Schools that do not have an individual consultant can call the local health department.

Since the symptoms of food poisoning (vomiting, stomach ache, and diarrhea) almost always occur within 24 hours of ingestion of the contaminated food, it is recommended that every school cafeteria routinely save, in the refrigerator, for 24 hours, a tray of food from every meal every day. If an outbreak occurs, this food can then be analyzed for toxic bacteria.

BURNS

Figure 16–20 shows the normal layers of skin.

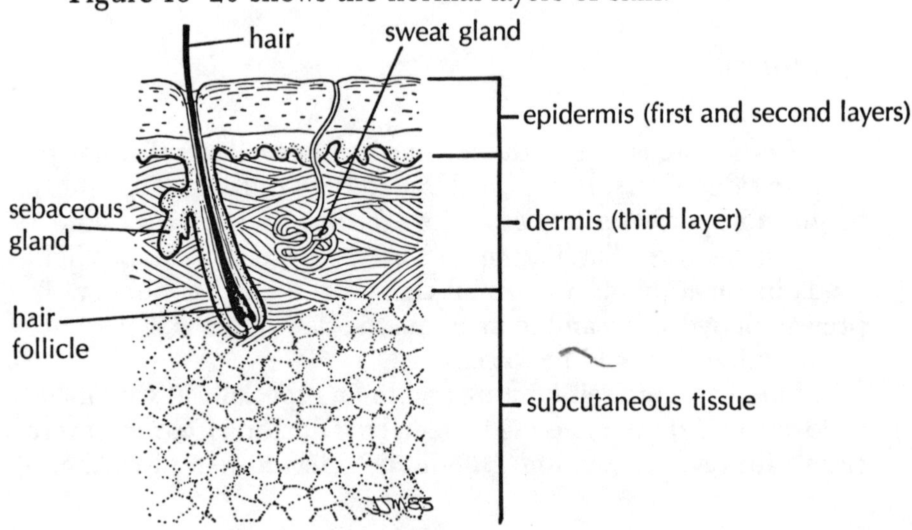

Figure 16–20. Normal layers of skin.

Nature of the Condition and Classification

First degree—redness with no blisters. Mild sunburn is a good example. This involves only the upper part of the first layer.

Second degree—redness with blisters. Severe sunburn or hot liquid are the most common causes. This involves the first and second layers of skin.

Third degree—at least the entire thickness of the skin and may include deeper muscles and even bone in severe burns such as occur in some explosions. The remaining skin tissues may be blanched white or charred black. There are usually no blisters; they have already broken.

Treatment

First degree. Relieve pain with cool compresses or anesthetic ointment (such as benzocain or lanacaine). Nothing else is necessary. Healing always occurs with no scar. As soon as the pain is gone, clean to prevent infection. A tiny burn can have an adhesive bandage applied. The child need not be sent home.

Second degree. Relieve pain with cool compresses, but gently so as not to break any blisters. If the blister can be kept intact, there will be no danger of infection until it eventually breaks, which blisters usually do within several days. A bulky padded bandage should be gently and loosely applied as a first aid measure after equally gentle cleaning with lukewarm water. The child should then see a physician for further treatment. The longer the blister remains intact, the more new skin will grow underneath, so that when the blister does break there will be less likelihood of infection and less pain from raw skin being exposed. A small second-degree burn on the arm or leg can be safely treated at school. It should be washed gently after waiting about 10 to 15 minutes for the pain to subside. Then, after gently patting dry, a small (4 inch by 4 inch) nonsticking gauze flat can be applied and held on with adhesive tape or gauze roller bandage. If in the judgment of the nurse or principal the circumstances are proper and the parent concurs, the child may stay at school but should not go out for recess or gym class for fear of injury to the new burn. Ointments are not harmful, but they moisten and weaken the blister and are conducive to breaking it. The only reason for applying ointment is to relieve pain; cool compresses do this better. Later, if infection is present, antibiotic ointments are necessary but should be prescribed by the physician.

Third degree. These burns are most apt to occur on direct exposure to flames, scalding liquids, or very hot metal. They represent a true medical emergency, not to be treated at school, and should be evacuated to the nearest hospital as quickly as possible. The burns should be covered loosely with a sheet or smooth towel. Ointments should not be applied.

INJURY TO INTERNAL ORGANS

Penetrating (Stab) Injury

Stab wounds of the chest or abdomen are extremely rare at most schools, the diagnosis is obvious, and there is never any doubt about what to do—immediate evacuation to the nearest hospital emergency room. If there is sufficient time, a large padded compression bandage may be applied, but not if it causes a delay in transfer to the hospital.

The parents should be notified after evacuation arrangements are made. If there is reason to suspect an ambulance will take more than a very few minutes, the school principal should take the initiative and have school personnel transport the child immediately.

Blunt Injury

Nature of the Condition

Injury to an internal organ from a nonpenetrating blow with a blunt object such as a rock, fist, or baseball bat is called a blunt injury. (See Figure 16–21.) There will be a bruise, large or small,

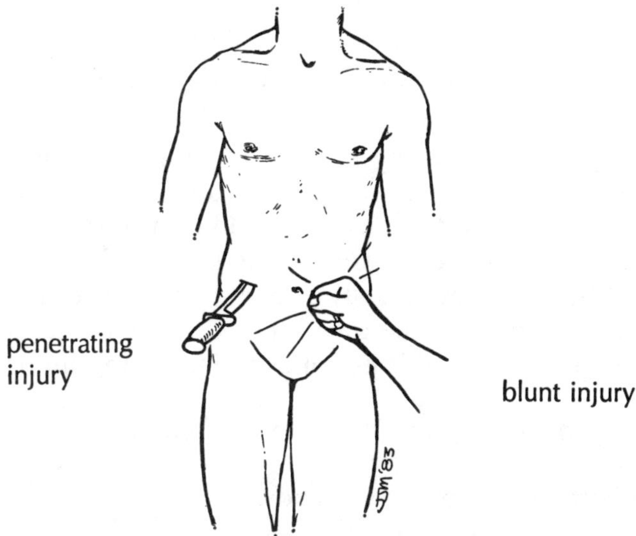

Figure 16–21. Penetrating and blunt injuries.

on the chest or abdomen where the child was struck, but the seriousness lies in the damage to the internal organ—the abdominal organ, heart, or lung.

Abdomen

A severe blow to the front of the abdomen can cause rupture or bleeding of the liver, spleen, stomach, or urinary bladder. A blow in the back may cause rupture of the kidneys. The initial blow will, of course, cause severe pain and often knock the wind out of the recipient of the blow. However, the initial symptoms may go away after a relatively short time, less than an hour in most cases. If there is no internal organ damage, no further symptoms will appear.

Rupture of an internal organ, however, can be very serious and may be missed if not suspected and watched for. The primary problem caused by a ruptured spleen or liver is bleeding into the abdominal cavity in large enough amounts to cause the child to go into a state of shock and die unless an operation is performed to tie off the bleeding blood vessels. If the stomach or urinary bladder is ruptured, the problem is compounded by toxic material escaping into the abdominal cavity causing peritonitis, which is apt to cause marked abdominal pain sooner.

Chest

The lungs or the heart may be damaged following a severe blow to the chest. There is no lengthy period between injury and onset of symptoms, usually less than ten minutes. The cause of the symptoms is usually the same as in abdominal organ injury—bleeding. In the chest the excess blood compresses the lung and/or heart, thus impeding their function. If the blow is severe enough, the lung may actually be torn by a fractured rib and then the escape of air from the torn lung adds to the difficulty. If this should happen, it would resemble a penetrating injury.

Symptoms of Blunt Injury to Abdominal Organ

1. History of blow to the abdomen
2. Apparent recovery in relatively short time
3. Gradual onset, two to six hours later, of symptoms of shock: weakness, dizziness, sweating, rapid weak pulse and respiration, gradual loss of consciousness, dilated pupils of the eye, deepening unconsciousness leading to coma and death.

Symptoms of Blunt Injury to Chest (Lung or Heart)

1. Rapid respiration
2. Extreme apprehension and fright from not being able to catch breath
3. Blueness around the lips
4. Rapid pulse
5. Gradual loss of consciousness in severe cases

Treatment

1. Observe child in clinic for 20 to 30 minutes.
2. Place in position of comfort.
3. If no further symptoms appear, allow child to go to class.
4. Check with teacher in one or two hours.
5. A ruptured stomach or bladder will usually result from a very severe blow, and the pain will be so severe that the

child obviously needs immediate medical attention by a physician.

6. Blunt injuries to internal organs result from blows of more than average severity. (See Figure 16–22.) Suspicious observation is necessary to alert one to the possibility. Delays in diagnosis are made when the child fails to report the accident or if the possibility is not considered at all.

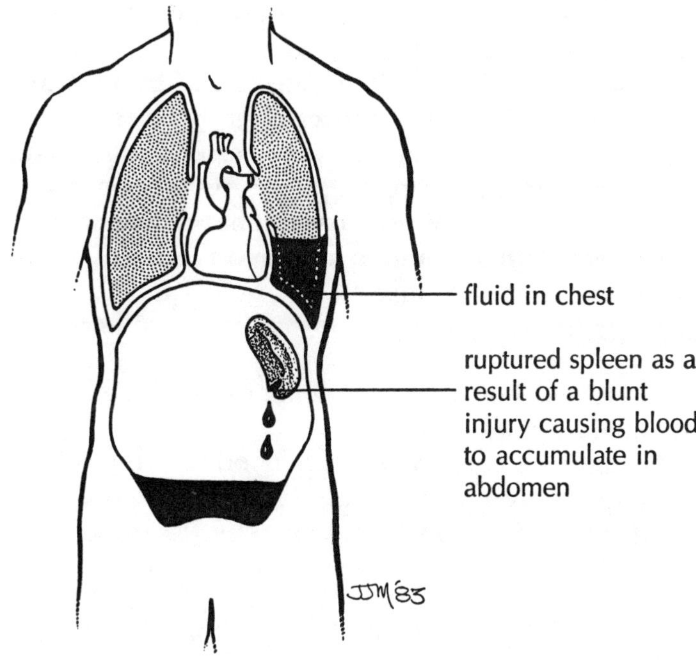

Figure 16–22. Fluid or blood in chest and/or abdomen.

HEAD INJURIES

Nature of the Condition

Head injuries are classified into bruises of the scalp, skull fractures, and damage to the brain itself.

A bruise of the scalp is caused by a light blow that usually causes no skull fracture, brain damage, or loss of consciousness. A characteristic and mildly painful *hematoma* ("goose egg" or "pump knot") is seen. (See Figure 16–23.) Ice is the best treatment; pressure is not necessary. If there is no concussion or loss of consciousness, no further treatment is necessary. The swelling usually lasts several days.

Skull fractures are of two principal varieties: linear and depressed. Linear fractures look, on x ray, like a cracked egg shell with both edges occupying about the same level as before the fracture. (See Figure 16–24.) They are caused by a relatively mild blow to the head. The blow causes pain, but the fracture itself heals with no special treatment. A depressed skull fracture does not mean the patient is depressed; it means a fragment of bone is pressing down on the brain such as might occur if someone were hit on the head with a hammer. This is very serious and requires urgent treatment. (See Figure 16–25.)

Damage to the brain itself is classified as follows:

1. *Laceration.* This is an actual cut or crushing injury, always accompanied by skull fractures.

2. *Contusion.* A rupture of small blood vessels inside the brain occurs. The leakage of blood destroys the surrounding brain tissue and is usually accompanied by skull fracture.

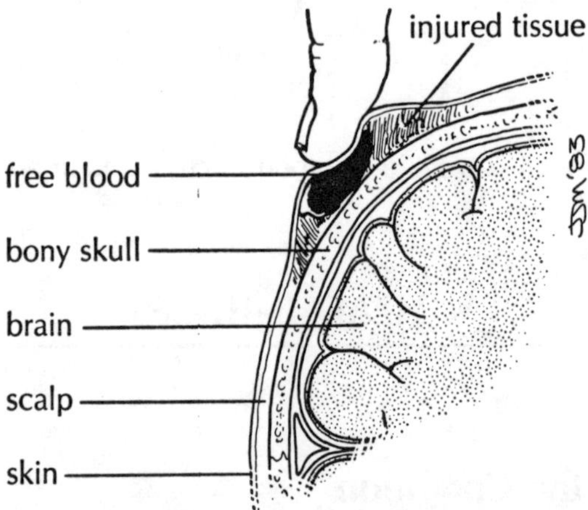

Figure 16–23. Hematoma of scalp. (The free blood under the skin feels soft and mushy. The injured tissue is swollen and hard, and a ridge can be felt (indicated by finger). This is often mistaken for a depressed skull fracture.)

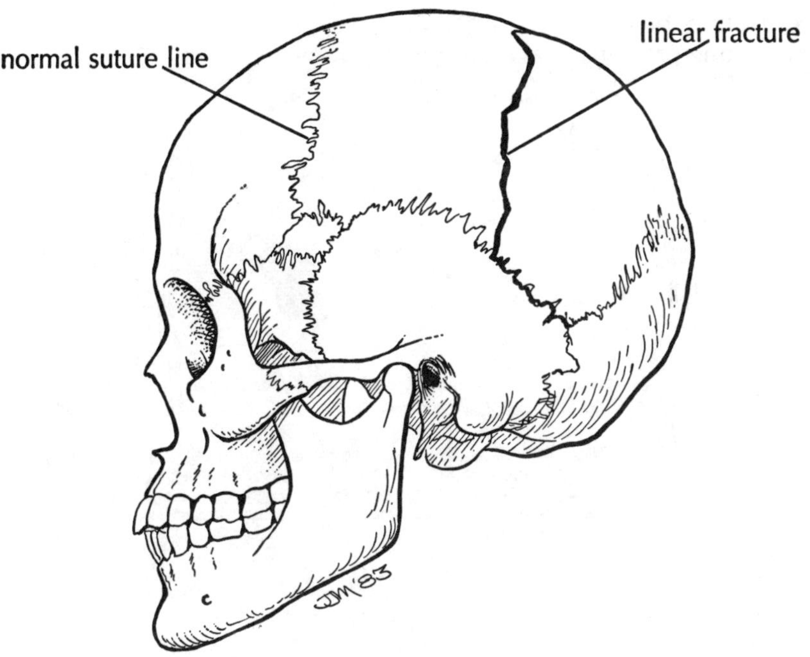

Figure 16–24. Linear skull fracture.

Both contusion and laceration result from severe head injury, are accompanied by loss of consciousness, and are never treated at school. Both require immediate evacuation to the nearest hospital emergency room.

3. *Concussion.* Of the three types of brain injury, this is the least severe. When a football player or a boxer "sees stars" or "has his bell rung," he has suffered a concussion. A concussion can be very mild, requiring only a short rest period, or it can be quite severe, requiring a day or two of rest in bed. If one were able to look at the brain after a mild concussion, nothing would be seen. The symptoms are caused by the brain being "shaken up."

Symptoms of Concussion

Severe

Loss of consciousness is the most important of all symptoms and must be assessed most carefully. If the student is deeply unconscious and cannot be awakened, it indicates a severe con-

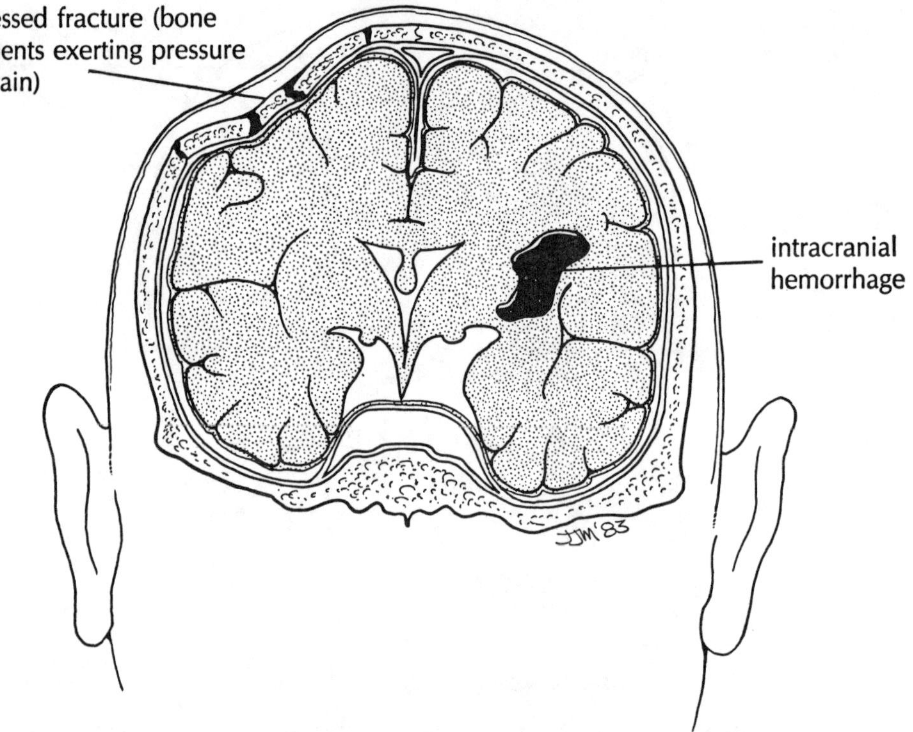

Figure 16–25. Depressed skull fracture with intracranial hemorrhage.

cussion. The more dilated the pupils, the more severe the concussion. Unequal pupils also have a serious import. At first the pulse and respiration may be rapid, but with deepening unconsciousness they will become slower. (See Figure 16–26.) Vomiting always indicates a more severe concussion. There can be loss of memory for recent events on awakening (*retrograde amnesia*).

Mild

A brief period of dizziness and/or disorientation occurs. There is a quick return to normality—the child may or may not remember what happened.

Diagnosis

A scalp bruise is diagnosed by inspection. Skull fracture can only be diagnosed by x ray. Brain contusion and lacerations follow

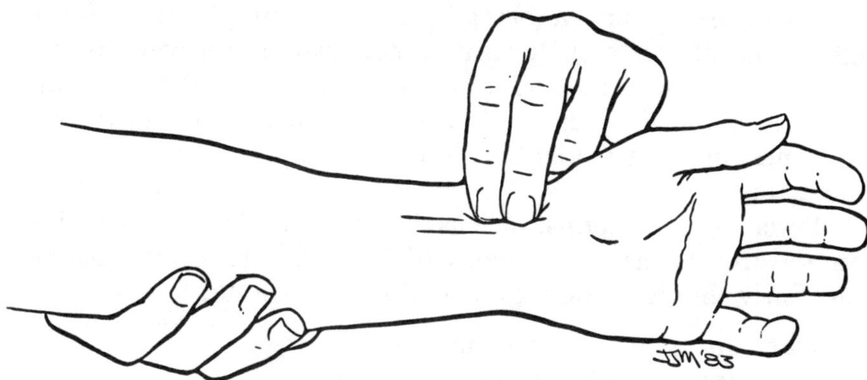

Figure 16–26. Taking the pulse.

severe head injury and will always be evacuated to a hospital for diagnosis. Concussion must always be strongly suspected following any blow to the head that causes momentary confusion, dizziness, or temporary unconsciousness.

Treatment

Concussion is the only important head injury that frequently requires school treatment. The cardinal principal of treatment is to prevent further injury to the head by an *absolute prohibition of further physical activity for the rest of the day;* in more severe concussion, as the doctor orders. It is well known that a second concussion soon after the first often leads to much more serious brain injury. The student should lie quietly for a few minutes with the head slightly elevated, and if it is a mild concussion, may then be allowed to sit. If the child remains asymptomatic, he or she may go back to class with a warning to the teacher to be alert.

Students with more severe concussion with a measurable period of unconsciousness should be evaluated by a physician.

Parents should always be notified in all types of concussion.

School Relevance

Normally, a mild concussion will cause no special problem; the child will rest and be perfectly normal later. There is, however, one notable exception—a football game. It is quite common for a high school player to suffer a mild concussion and continue to play, either because the student doesn't report it to the coach or trainer or because, if reported, it is not regarded with sufficient seriousness and the student is allowed to play again during that same game.

Several organizations, such as the American Medical Association and the American Academy of Pediatrics, have formulated some fairly simple guidelines that all schools should follow:

One concussion—out of the game
Two concussions—out for the season
Three concussions—out for school career

This would prevent many deaths from head injuries, which occur every year in the United States during secondary school athletic contests.

INTRACRANIAL HEMORRHAGE

Nature of the Condition

On occasion, a blow to the head will cause rupture of a blood vessel between the brain and bony skull without causing any direct damage to the brain tissue or skull fracture. This is very serious because blood can collect rapidly and cause deeper and deeper unconsciousness from continually increasing pressure on the brain. (See Figure 16–27.)

Symptoms and Diagosis

All of the symptoms listed under concussion may be present.

There is one special type of intracranial hemorrhage, called *subdural* or *epidural bleeding,* which is characterized by a relatively

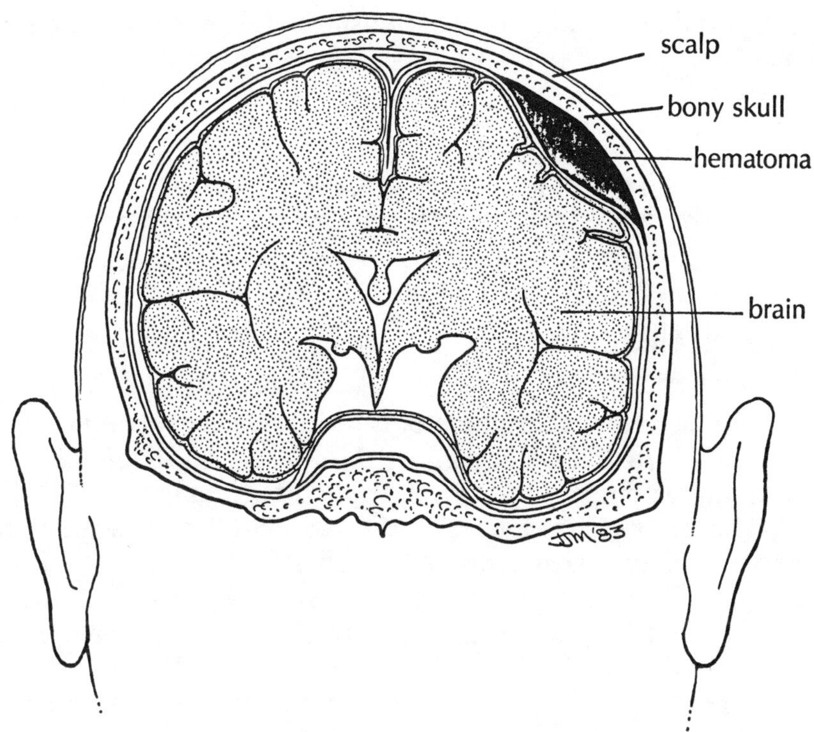

Figure 16–27. Subdural hematoma. (There is no skull fracture or brain damage. The blood collects as a result of a blow on the head, which causes rupture of small blood vessels.)

brief period of unconsciousness followed by awakening and seeming normality. Several hours or days later, however, because of continued but slow bleeding, the student may exhibit unusual behavior or slowly lapse into unconsciousness again. This double period of unconsciousness has grave implications.

Treatment and Role of the School Nurse

Any child who is "knocked out" should be evaluated by the symptoms listed under severe and mild concussion. Any of the severe symptoms indicate a need for medical evaluation right away, not at the end of the school day.

A double period of unconsciousness also requires immediate evacuation.

TEMPERATURE MEASUREMENT

Types of Thermometers

The electronic thermometer is relatively new, very quick, and accurate. It can save time when used for large groups of children. It is quite expensive—this is the major disadvantage.

The glass thermometer is the old standby. It is accurate, inexpensive, and most commonly used.

Recently, plastic or paper strips have become available to place on the forehead. Some can be used several times, and some are for single use. They have two disadvantages. If they are used for large groups of children, the total cost can be great. Second, they have not proved to be very accurate and, at this time, are not recommended.

Feeling the forehead is the traditional method. Though doctors have urged thermometer use for decades, parents will probably continue to rely on their sense of touch. *This is the most inaccurate method of all,* especially for children with serious illnesses such as appendicitis or diphtheria that typically begin with a low-grade fever.

Normal Temperature

There is no single level of "normal" body temperature. The traditional glass thermometer has an arrow at 98.6 degrees Fahrenheit because the majority of people in temperate climates have under-tongue temperature readings of about 98.2 to 99 degrees. In actuality, a child's (or adult's) body temperature normally varies from low in the morning to high in the late afternoon and evening. An average healthy person's oral temperature will usually be about 96 to 97 degrees shortly after awakening in the morning and gradually go up to 98 to 99 degrees in the afternoon. Many perfectly normal individuals have an afternoon temperature of 99.6 to 100 degrees, especially in hot summer climates. (See Figure 16–28.)

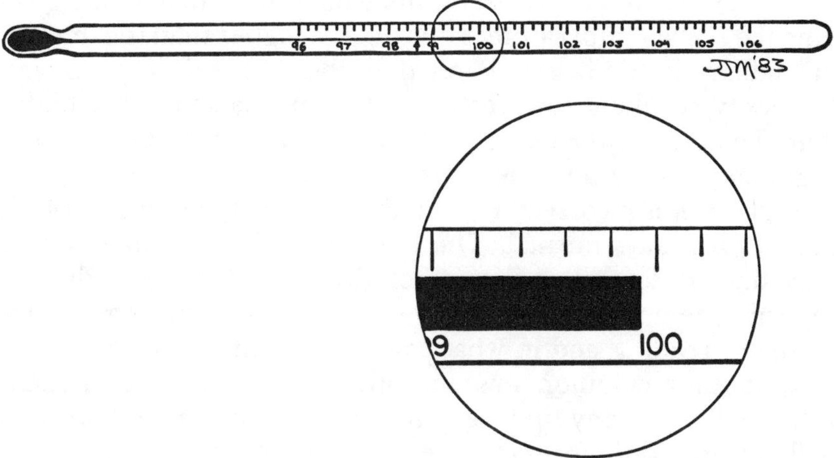

Figure 16–28. Temperature just under 100 degrees

Fever

In order to determine if a child has fever, meaning an abnormal temperature elevation, one must know that child's normal body temperature for that time of the day. Since this is rarely known beforehand, a temperature between 99 and 100 degrees may or may not constitute fever for that individual child. Therefore, unless a child has some other symptoms of illness, doctors are apt to regard an oral temperature of 100 degrees or less as only a possible sign of illness and suggest that the child be watched closely for further symptoms.

Temperature readings over 100 degrees usually indicate some type of infection, though there are a small number of normal individuals with no illness at all but a temperature of 100 to 100.6 degrees. Readings of 101 degrees or over are always abnormal and are to be considered as fever.

Methods of Measurement

The usual methods of temperature measurement are oral, rectal, and axillary (armpit). The first two are more reliable; the axillary temperature varies more with changes in air temperature.

There is an old rule of thumb which states that at any given time the rectal temperature is one degree higher than the oral and the axillary is one degree lower than the oral. *This is not accurate.* Generally speaking, the rectal temperature is somewhat higher than the oral and the axillary is lower, but it is practically never an exact one degree and there are times when they are the same. Therefore, it is incorrect to think that a rectal temperature of 100 degrees is always normal. The level of the body temperature is only one of several indicators of disease. When recording or reporting temperature, one should always state the actual thermometer reading and in what part of the body it was measured.

Another common misconception is that the thermometer with the long skinny tip is only for oral use and the one with the bulbous tip is only for rectal use. With proper cleansing, they can be used interchangeably.

Time of Measurement

The number of minutes the thermometer should be left in place varies with the type of thermometer used, but most instructional pamphlets suggest leaving it in place about three minutes; this is usually longer than necessary. In most cases, the thermometer will reach its peak in about one minute. It is easy enough to take the thermometer out after one minute, read it, reinsert it, and read it after another minute. In most cases the reading will be seen to be the same or 0.2 to 0.4 of a degree higher. Using this method, the school nurse or clinic aide learns how long the thermometer must be left in place and saves time and some discomfort for the child.

Factors causing misleading temperature readings include:

1. Excessive environmental heat and humidity
2. Excessive exposure to cold
3. Excessive physical exercise

4. Decreased air circulation
5. Recent eating or drinking of hot or cold foods
6. A child sneaking the thermometer under the hot water faucet because he or she wants to go home

HEAT-RELATED ILLNESS

Nature of the Condition

There are four types of adverse physical reactions to excess heat and humidity. The higher the humidity, the more dangerous is a high air temperature because of decreased evaporation of body sweat. Exercise causes increased sweating and body metabolism which leads to greater loss of body water and/or electrolyte (sodium, potassium etc.). If these losses are severe, the adverse reactions may vary from simple fainting to fatal heat stroke. This can occur indoors and in climates that are not excessively hot.

Symptoms

1. *Heat syncope.* This is simple fainting or near fainting caused by overheating. It begins with dizziness, usually while the student is standing or running. The blood pressure goes down and the body (rectal) temperature is high—103 to 105 degrees Fahrenheit. The skin is usually moist.

2. *Heat cramps.* Tightening, cramps, and spasms of active muscles occur, usually during intense, prolonged exercise in hot weather. There is no loss of consciousness. This is associated with low body sodium.

3. *Heat exhaustion.* The early symptoms are dizziness, weakness, exhaustion, nausea, and vomiting. The student may become irrational and belligerent. There may be associated muscle cramps. The rectal temperature is high. The skin is flushed and usually moist, but in extreme cases it can be dry. If the symptoms

continue, partial or complete unconsciousness may ensue and lead to heat stroke.

4. *Heat stroke.* This is an acute medical emergency with extremely high fever, 106 to 108 degrees Fahrenheit, disorientation, twitching, seizures, and coma. The skin is hot and dry.

Heat-related illnesses are usually not seen as clearly separate entities; they often merge into each other, especially if proper treatment is delayed. For example, there may be doubt about heat exhaustion versus impending heat stroke. *Whenever there is doubt, always suspect the worst.*

Treatment

Heat syncope, heat cramps, and heat exhaustion are all treated by rest, placement in a cool, shaded area, replacement of water by drinking, and cooling of the skin with cold water and/or a fan. This is usually sufficient.

Heavy clothing should be loosened or removed and resumption of exercise should be delayed for at least two to three hours.

Children who experience more severe symptoms such as irrationality or partial loss of consciousness should be evaluated by their physician.

If heat stroke occurs, oral fluids can rarely be swallowed. Rapid evacuation to a medical emergency room is mandatory but at the same time the skin should be cooled with water, ice, and/or a fan. If available, oxygen should be given.

Prevention

All heat-related illness is preventable if proper measures are taken.

1. Exercise preconditioning, heat acclimatization, and water replacement are the most important factors.
2. Lightweight, loose, cool clothing should be worn.
3. Athletes are at special risk and occasionally require enforced extra water intake.

4. Cool or cold water should be available since it is absorbed more quickly from the stomach.
5. Salt and/or calcium tablets are of no benefit. If enough water is drunk, the body automatically conserves salt and calcium, so it is not necessary to give tablets.
6. Commercial electrolyte solutions are not harmful and may be used if desired. They are no more effective than water.
7. Students who sweat a lot should salt their food more liberally.
8. Predisposing conditions that make a child more likely to develop heat illness are as follows:
   a. Cystic fibrosis
   b. Vomiting or diarrhea
   c. Fever from any cause, even an immunization
   d. Obesity
   e. Voluntary water restriction
   f. Poor acclimatization
   g. Prior heat-related illness

Role of the School Nurse

If no qualified athletic trainers are available, the school nurse's expertise may be lifesaving. The following factors are to be considered:

1. Plenty of cool water should be available for athletes during all game and practice sessions.
2. Athletes who lose more than three percent of their body weight (about 5 to 7 pounds for a 200 pound athlete) because of sweat loss during a practice session, are at special risk. An accurate scale should be available.
3. Athletic personnel should be alerted to the possible dangers of excess salt tablets causing high-sodium dehydration. High water intake is much more efficient in maintaining good fluid and electrolyte balance.
4. All personnel should be cautioned about the dangers of voluntary water deprivation to produce weight loss, especially in athletes.
5. A copy of the *Sports Medicine Guide* and the *School Health Guide,* both published by the American Academy of Pedi-

atrics contains additional useful information. They can be ordered from P.O. Box 1034, Evanston, IL, 60201.

CARDIOPULMONARY RESUSCITATION (CPR)

School Relevance and Role of the School Nurse

CPR is now the accepted method of lifesaving. Many school districts offer, and some mandate, CPR training to school nurses, secretaries, cafeteria managers, teachers, coaches, athletic trainers, and principals. Athletic trainers and some nurses receive CPR training during their course work leading to certification and licensing.

The school nurse is the person people will instinctively turn to in a medical emergency and therefore is the logical person to be trained in CPR basic life support. However, if the nurse is not on campus daily, it is best to also train someone who is. If the school nurse is selected to be a CPR instructor, it will require a great deal of time out of an already busy schedule and will require the hiring of additional staff.

Levels of Training

The American Heart Association and the American Red Cross have taken the lead in establishing training courses throughout the United States. There are three levels of training and expertise, depending on the time spent in training, teaching, and actually doing CPR.

1. Resuscitators are persons trained in basic life support. This requires 4 to 8 hours of training which must be renewed annually.
2. Instructors are qualified to teach basic life support. This requires the basic course plus 16 additional hours of

training. In addition, a course must be taught at least once a year.

3. Instructor-trainers are qualified to teach instructors. They must have the same qualifications as instructors and are then selected individually by the program director.

Resuscitation Methods

Detailed CPR instruction is available in many books, booklets, and pamphlets; some very detailed. This discussion will be limited to the main methods of CPR available and when it should and should not be used.

Mouth-to-Mouth Resuscitation

Mouth-to-mouth resuscitation should *only* be attempted if there has been a cessation of breathing and a patient is making no respiratory efforts on his or her own. As soon as spontaneous breathing starts, the rescuer should stop so as not to hinder the patient's own breathing efforts.

Chest Compression

When the patient's heart has completely stopped and no pulse can be felt in the neck, upper arm or wrist, and the patient is unconscious, proper, intermittent chest compression will keep the blood in circulation. This may keep body cells alive (especially brain cells) until the heart resumes its own spontaneous beat.

Back Blows, Heimlich Hug, Finger Sweep of Throat

Airway obstruction is often caused by a bolus of food, usually a piece of meat. Children may choke on peanuts or popcorn. The patient grasps the front of the throat, cannot speak, turns blue, and rapidly loses consciousness. Coughing is not present.

The Heimlich Hug and sharp blows to the back are both recommended; the Hug to rapidly expel the foreign object, and the back blows to dislodge it if the Hug doesn't work.

If neither of the above works, the finger sweep is a method of thrusting a curled finger into the back of the throat to manually remove the obstructing object.

Cautions

1. All methods of CPR require previous training and practice on a mannikin—never on another person.
2. A person who is coughing should be left alone to cough up whatever is causing the cough.
3. Any person who is making respiratory efforts should be left alone.
4. If the heart is beating, chest compression should not be attempted.
5. The material in this brief section is not to be considered a substitute for CPR training and complete illustrated handbooks; it is merely a brief summary for school personnel who may have no other immediate resource. An excellent small, practical, reference manual is *How to Save a Life Using CPR* by Lindsay R. Curtis, M.D. It is available from H.P. Books, P.O. Box 5367, Tucson, AZ 85703.

SECTION 17

SEVERE PHYSICAL HANDICAPS

This section describes the situation of children with severe physical handicaps in schools since the passage of Public Law 94–142 and provides specific information and guidelines for treatment of two such handicaps—spina bifida and mental retardation.

PUBLIC LAW 94–142

Since the passage in 1972 of Public Law (PL) 94–142, Education for All Handicapped Children, there has been a concerted effort to enroll as many handicapped children as possible in the regular school system, public and private. School systems plus groups outside the school system—parents, doctors, cerebral palsy associations, lawyers, physiotherapists, occupational therapists, and others—have contributed to the effort.

In past years, most parents of children with severe physical handicaps were advised to keep them home, keep them clean, and not try to teach them very much. Most children with cerebral palsy were regarded by parents and doctors alike as mentally retarded as well as palsied. With experience and better understanding, it has become apparent that various kinds of education and training are indeed beneficial. There is no longer any doubt that handicapped children belong in a school setting. They are immeasurably happier, and there is no question that they make greater advances in self-help and other skills than when they stay home. Many schools have proved exceptionally successful in providing education for many handicapped children from kindergarten through high school, and many who have graduated become partly or fully independent adults.

Obviously, most handicapped children can manage fairly well in a regular mainstream class. However, because of pressures that have arisen since passage of PL 94–142, some severely handicapped children are being placed in an untenable and unhappy classroom situation (regular mainstream class) that is not good for them now nor is it good for their future life adjustment. One must face reality; a child with moderate to severe cerebral palsy, for example, is never going to be "normal." True, that child is going to have to live with normal people, but the proper time for integration with those normal people is certainly not at ages three to six. This child's brain has the same capacity for hopes, fears, disappointments, and desires for acceptance as exist in all other children of that age, even though he or she is unable to communicate or play with peers. It is a developmental period during which all children have very little insight into themselves or the distresses of others. These feelings of empathy normally come later in life, beginning in preadolescence and coming to full fruition in normal, full adolescent development. Therefore, the severely handicapped child needs a certain amount of support and protection from normal peers until a little later in life. At that time, tentative trials can determine whether or not the child is ready for mainstreaming in a regular class on a regular campus. The school nurse should be aware that the desire of the parents for their children to be as near normal as possible is so strong that there may be disagreement over the child's placement. With medical and nursing expertise, the school nurse is in an excellent position to mediate disputes and help parents and school personnel decide on proper class placement.

SPINA BIFIDA

Nature of the Condition

Spina bifida—or *myelomeningocoele*—is a failure of the vertebral bones (spinal column) to fuse, leaving the enclosed spinal cord unprotected. While this may occur anywhere from the neck to the tail bone, the most common location is the lower part of the spine just above the buttocks. In addition, the skin and spinal cord do not develop properly, and a pouch varying in size from a walnut to a grapefruit often is present where the bones fail to fuse. (See Figure 17–1.) This pouch contains all of the nerves of the spinal cord that are supposed to go to the lower pelvis and legs. In a typical case, the child has no control over bowel or bladder and both legs are completely paralyzed.

Hydrocephalus (water on the brain) is often associated with spina bifida. This can be prevented or controlled with proper treatment.

In children with a large pouch, the skin is often very thin and may leak spinal fluid. This can also be surgically corrected.

Spina bifida occulta (hidden spina bifida) is a condition in which the failure of fusion of the lower spinal vertebrae is slight, and there is no outpouching of the skin, and there are very little

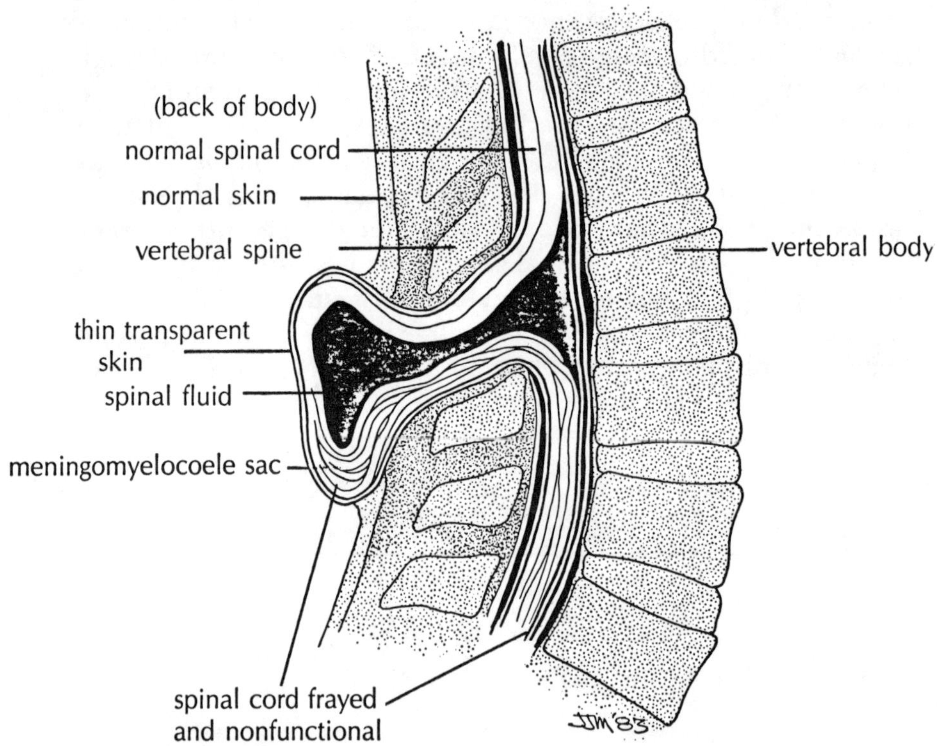

Figure 17–1. Myelomeningocoele. (The spinal fluid completely surrounds the spinal cord and is immediately below the skin of the sac. The skin consists only of a thin membrane, which often ruptures spontaneously.)

or no spinal nerve abnormalities. In most cases there are no bladder or bowel symptoms or leg involvement.

Unless there are associated abnormalities of the brain, and usually there are not, children with spina bifida are emotionally and intellectually normal. With proper treatment and training, they should be able to attend school. Indeed, there are now many children with properly treated spina bifida attending school in regular classes with normal children. They have excellent potential for learning.

Spina bifida associations exist in many large cities. Parents of these children, like parents of all handicapped children, have special needs, and organizations of this nature are very helpful.

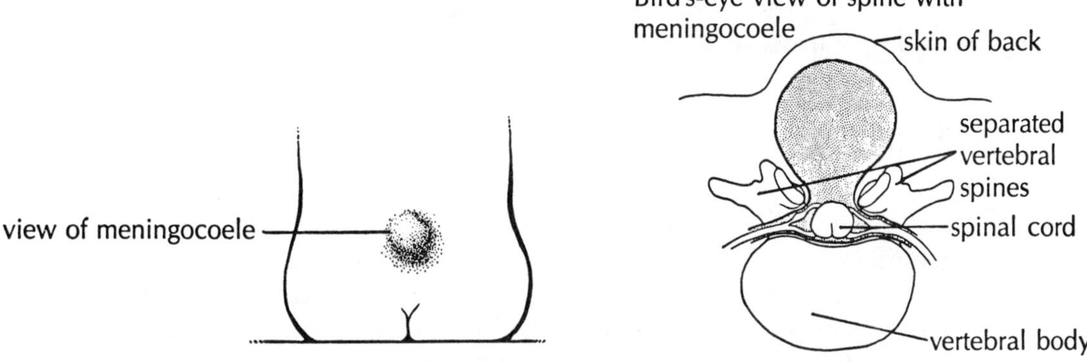

Figure 17–2. Meningocoele. (The meninges or sac that contains the spinal fluid is pouched out between the separated vertebral spines, but the spinal cord itself is normal. The skin is of near normal thickness. The person has little to no paralysis and may have normal bladder and bowel functions.)

Diagnosis and Symptoms

Because of the size of the pouch, the diagnosis is usually made at birth. There are rare cases in which the bones almost completely fuse and the visible pouch is very small. In these cases the nerve damage may be slight, and the resulting bowel or bladder or leg paralysis problem may also be slight. (See Figure 17–2.) In cases of this nature, urinary or fecal incontinence or clumsiness in walking may be noticeable, and the child should be referred to a physician for evaluation.

Spina bifida occulta often causes no symptoms whatsoever. Symptoms such as enuresis, bowel problems, or sensory or motor lower extremity problems may be caused by a variety of other conditions and must be referred to a physician for diagnosis and initiation of treatment. About 20 percent of all children who, for unrelated reasons, receive x-rays of the lower spine will show a tiny failure of the closure of the vertebral bones. Some of these children will also have enuresis or encopresis (bowel soiling). Many years ago this type of spina bifida occulta was thought to be a cause of bed wetting. Currently, most authorities feel there is no cause-and-effect relationship between this incidental x-ray finding and a urinary or fecal problem.

In questionable cases, an investigation by a neurologist or urologist must be made.

Treatment

Primary treatment is always surgical. Since this condition is so complicated and has medical, social, and educational aspects, the entire treatment team must include a pediatrician, a neurosurgeon, a urologist, an orthopedist, a social worker, an occupational therapist, and a physical therapist, as well as the school nurse.

Surgical treatment will generally center around one or all of three major procedures, which will already have been done by the time the child starts school:

1. Repair of the skin defect in the lower back
2. Shunt-type procedures in the brain to prevent or arrest hydrocephalus
3. Orthopedic procedures to the legs to enable the child to walk with braces and crutches at an appropriate time

However, even after school attendance begins, medical consultation and some surgical procedures may be necessary throughout the patient's lifetime.

School Relevance and Role of the School Nurse

A typical spina bifida child of school age will already have had back surgery to repair the skin defect, a shunt in the brain to prevent or arrest hydrocephalus, and braces and crutches for walking. In addition, many children require diapers and diaper changes for fecal and/or urinary incontinence.

The school nurse may be asked to monitor and consult with the physician in the following areas:

1. *Skin of the lower back.* Usually very little care is required. Occasionally, however, the scar may become infected, become dry and itchy, or develop crusts. Treatment is to remove crusts gently,

apply antibiotic ointment if necessary for infection, cleanse with antibacterial soap, or occasionally apply softening lotions.

2. *Bowel care.* Because of lack of muscular control of the anal opening, fecal soiling is often seen. Changes of diapers or other appropriate clothing must be kept at school. Privacy and due regard for the child's sensitivities are absolutely essential.

3. *Bladder care.* Because of lack of nerve supply to the bladder, the urge to urinate does not exist. Therefore, the bladder fills till it can hold no more, and eventually urine dribbles out of the urethra and keeps the clothes or diaper constantly wet. Since the bladder never empties, the remaining urine and bladder wall always becomes infected. Modern management requires that the bladder be emptied periodically to prevent infection. Some older children have learned to empty their bladders by lower abdominal pressure, but most urologists feel that intermittent catheterization every four to six hours is the preferred method. Many school nurses now perform this procedure. It is usually performed once a day at school at about noon. Close contact and consultation must be maintained between school nurse, parent, and physician. Usually school nurses will require a little extra in-service training if they have not performed this procedure for a long time, but the technique is quite simple and can be learned (or relearned) in a short time. Many urologists teach young children self-catheterization. The age at which children can do this varies depending on individual ability, but is usually between five and seven years. In these cases, the school nurse should work closely with the principal to provide the space and privacy and to make other necessary arrangements.

4. *Care of the legs, braces, and crutches.* The school nurse should be aware of possible pressure sores from braces. Sometimes, extra padding may be necessary. Occasionally, notification to the parents or physician for an adjustment will be necessary. Observation of the child while walking will reveal whether the crutches are of proper length and the child is using them properly.

5. *Observation of head size.* A child with spina bifida should be brought into the clinic each month to have head circumference recorded on the health card. Though there may be an intracranial shunt, its valves occasionally malfunction. Therefore, any unusual head growth—more than ½ inch in six months—should be reported to the parent and/or physician.

6. *Class placement and learning problems.* Most spina bifida children can be mainstreamed into regular classes. Many, however, have specific learning problems and poor fine motor control because of subtle cerebral defects, also called perceptual problems. Therefore, psychometric evaluations may be helpful in preparing an individual educational plan (IEP).

7. *Special problems at adolescence.* As would be expected, depression frequently occurs. Girls worry about child bearing and boys worry about potency. Normal experiences with children of the opposite sex are lacking. Most adolescents need to know more about their condition; their parents have been told but they haven't. The school nurse and school counselor can be most helpful. A peer group rap session with other handicapped and normal children may give an adolescent an opportunity to express his or her anxieties.

MENTAL RETARDATION

Nature of the Condition

There are two major categories of mental retardation—high-level and low-level. The diagnostic nomenclature varies from state to state. Also, medical designations are sometimes different from educational designations.

High-Level

In the recent past many school systems designated children with an IQ between 70 and 85 or 90 as "educable mentally retarded." Some school systems still do. The educational diagnosis is made from the scores on the IQ test and ability to learn basic academic material—reading, writing, spelling, and arithmetic.

Health specialists and some psychologists are reluctant to make a diagnosis of mental retardation at this high level, because observation of this type of child over long periods of time has shown that about two-thirds of them become normal adults; they marry, work, raise children, and function the same as adults who were not so categorized when they were young school children.

Low-Level

Children with measured IQ scores of about 50 to 70 are sometimes called "trainable mentally retarded" or mentally defec tive. There is little to no disagreement about the diagnosis; both educational and medical specialists usually agree.

The American Association for Mental Deficiency has developed an official classification system that is based on the degree of mental and physical retardation. The higher-level children in this category have an IQ of about 50 to 70; the best example is a child with mongolism, or Down's Syndrome. The lowest level in this category is the child who is physically and mentally retarded to such a severe degree that he or she is completely bedridden, must be tube fed, and gives no indication of any awareness of his or her surroundings. This type of child acquires no self-help skills and requires complete custodial care.

Diagnosis and Symptoms

High-Level

There are no overt symptoms or signs. Academic performance and IQ testing are the only diagnostic clues. On casual observation the child looks, acts, speaks, and understands about as well as other children. Physical ability is usually normal or close to normal. However, first to third grade school work is performed very poorly, if at all. Brain functions most seriously affected are memory, spatial relationships, and sequencing ability—those functions most likely to affect learning of basic academic material.

The medical background is usually normal. Walking and talking usually begin at a normal age, as do tricycle riding and toilet training. Socialization with peers at ages three, four, and five is usually normal.

Most parents of children in this category see their children as normal in all respects until they start school. This is why it is so difficult for a parent to accept a diagnosis of mental retardation in a child of this nature. Indeed, public pressure against this diagnosis has finally led many school systems to discard the category from their classifications for special children. Also, the score on an IQ test has been criticized as being much too restrictive as a sole measure of intelligence. In many ways, the IQ test is simply another achievement test rather than a test of anything innate. Provided all other factors are equal, a child who grows up in a nurturing, reading family will perform better (score higher) on an IQ test than that same child would if he or she grew up in a nonnurturing, nonreading environment.

Low-Level

There are many signs and symptoms. The medical or developmental history reveals delays in many functions, motor as well as cognitive. Crawling and walking occur late. Language comprehension is poor from a very early age, and spoken language may never develop at all.

The incidence of convulsive seizures is much higher than in the normal population.

The facial appearance is often abnormal. In many cases the features are broad and thick, the mouth often remains open, and the brow is narrow. The ears may be low-set or unusually shaped. In medical jargon, these abnormalities are called *stigmata.*

Many identified syndromes are associated with chromosomal or metabolic abnormalities plus mental retardation. These syndromes usually have two or three names, one after the individual who first described it and another that is descriptive of the disorder. Dr. John L. H. Down first described the condition, characterized in part by a peculiar eye configuration, hence the term *mongolism.* Other characteristics are short, stubby fingers and a peculiar crease in the palm of the hand. In the past 20 years it has been discovered that the number 21 chromosome has three parts instead of the normal two, so that now the disease is sometimes referred to as trisomy–21. There are more than 100 well-defined syndromes associated with low-level mental retardation. More are discovered and described each year. (See Bergsma's *Birth Defects Compendium.*)

Treatment

High-Level

As a group, these children are physically and emotionally normal. They have no increased susceptibility to disease and need no special care. They can participate in all school activity.

Low-Level

A great deal of nursing care is necessary in this group of children; the amount depends on the degree of retardation.

Children who are high on the scale of low-level retardation can usually be trained to feed themselves and handle their own toilet needs; however, they usually need help until they are beyond six years of age.

Because of poor personal hygiene, the incidence of impetigo is higher.

The incidence of impacted ear wax is much higher in mentally retarded children. It is rarely serious enough to interfere with hearing, but as the wax continues to collect, it should be irrigated and washed out periodically. The child can be referred to a physician, or the school nurse, if properly trained, can perform this function. If school nurses are to perform this procedure, they must first learn to use an otoscope and demonstrate proficiency under supervision. The wax must first be softened with an appropriate solution and then irrigated with a gentle stream of water. In my experience a "water pic" does not exert enough pressure; a metal ear syringe works better. There are several ear-softening agents available. Two commonly used are Cerumenex® and Debrox®. Cerumenex is stronger, slightly irritating to the skin, and requires a prescription. It works better but should not be given to parents to use at home. It should be dropped into the ear, allowed to remain for 30 to 60 minutes, and then washed out. Debrox is completely nonirritating and does not require a prescription. The parent may use it at home for three to five days before the ear irrigation. In either case, the procedure may have to be repeated one or two times. If the child complains of pain, the procedure should be stopped and repeated two or three days later if a sizable amount of wax remains.

Mentally retarded children who have seizures tend to have them more frequently and more severely than nonretarded epileptic children. Some fall and hit their heads so often they must wear a protective football helmet at all times. The treatment is the same as described in the section on epilepsy. The incidence of *status epilepticus*, however, is significantly higher, so this group of children must be watched more closely.

School Relevance and Role of the School Nurse

Since handicapped children may be admitted to preschool programs at one to two years of age, there are two highly relevant questions that the school nurse will be asked.

Is the Child Contagious?

Babies born with congenital herpes simplex or congenital rubella (German measles) may be severely mentally retarded and may be contagious for varying periods of time. The virus can be found in various body secretions including saliva. These are the only forms of low-level mental retardation that pose any threat of contagion in school.

Babies with congenital rubella often shed virus for weeks or months but never years. By the age of three years, they are no longer contagious. If teachers or other school personnel must be near younger children with rubella, they might contract the disease. Therefore, they should be tested for susceptibility (a simple blood test) and immunized with rubella vaccine if necessary. This is especially true if the teacher is of childbearing age; rubella infection in the early months of pregnancy can lead to serious birth defects.

It takes about six weeks for the teacher to develop immunity after immunization. If a very young (under one year old) rubella baby is to be admitted to school, ample time must be allowed for all necessary school personnel to develop immunity after receiving the vaccine.

Pregnant women or women who could become pregnant in six weeks are cautioned not to receive the vaccine. It is a live virus vaccine and there is a possibility of the virus being transmitted to the fetus and causing congenital rubella. A serious dilemma may arise if the school has a special education program that admits very young babies and some of the teachers in that building are susceptible to rubella and may be pregnant or become pregnant. The solution to this dilemma is administrative. Homebound programs or teacher transfers are two options.

Herpes simplex virus may infect a fetus during pregnancy and cause severe brain damage. Some of these infants live for many years with severe physical and mental retardation, and some will be enrolled in public schools. If they have fever blisters around their mouths and noses, they are just as contagious as any normal child with the fever blisters of herpes simplex. However, since they must be handled more and since they often drool, the opportunity for spread of the virus is greater. Therefore, hand washing is more important. Also, the school nurse should set up certain techniques, procedures, and routines similar to those used in hospital contagious disease wards but adapted to school use.

The herpes virus in children with brain damage caused by congenital herpes acts the same way it does in normal children who contact herpes from friends. It lies dormant in the body and is only contagious when it becomes manifest as the familiar cold sore or fever blister seen around the mouth or nose.

Is the Disease Progressive; Is It Getting Worse?

The vast majority of children with severe mental deficiency have nonprogressive disease. The damage to the brain was suffered long before, and the infection or trauma is no longer present, although complications such as pneumonia and bed sores occur frequently and often lead to early death.

There are, however, rare diseases of the brain that lead to progressive and contagious brain damage. These diseases are often fatal. They are discussed in Section 7 under the heading "Progressive Diseases of the Nervous System." They are rarely, if ever, contagious. The role of the school nurse is simply to offer supportive nursing care as long as the child remains in school.

APPENDIX OF FORMS

The following forms are either direct examples or composites of forms actually in use in various schools. Many more exist. These are offered only as examples; school nurses will need to adapt them for use in their own school district and/or for their own personal use.

REPORTING FORM FOR STUDENTS ON MEDICATION FOR LEARNING OR BEHAVIOR PROBLEMS

Date of Report ________________

TO BE COMPLETED BY CAMPUS NURSE

Name __________ Birthdate ______________ School __________ Grade __________

Medication __________________________ Diagnosis __________________________

Dose schedule (All prescribed doses) AM: Home School Dose ☐ Noon: Home School Dose ☐ PM: Home School Dose ☐

Date began initially ______________________ Physician ______________________

Date began this school year ______________________________________

Adverse effects of medication: ☐ None ☐ Drowsiness ☐ Headache

☐ Loss of weight ☐ Weight gain ☐ Upset stomach ☐ Loss of appetite

☐ Hyperactivity worse ☐ Other (explain) ______________________

____
School Nurse

TO BE FILLED OUT BY CLASSROOM TEACHER

	Not at all	Just a little	Pretty much	Very much
1. Restless or overactive, excitable, impulsive				
2. Disturbs other children				
3. Fails to finish things started				
4. Short attention span				
5. Constant fidgeting				
6. Inattentive, easily distracted				
7. Demands must be met immediately				
8. Cries often and easily				
9. Mood changes quickly and drastically				
10. Temper outbursts, explosive and unpredictable behavior				

Conner's Abbreviated Behavior Rating Scale

____
Classroom Teacher

MEDICATION PERMISSION REQUEST FORM

Note to Parents/Guardians:

The ________________ independent School District requires that all students who need medication during school hours must do the following:

1. Present a written consent form signed by the parent or legal guardian.
2. Bring the medication in the original prescription bottle, properly labeled by a registered pharmacist as prescribed by law.

Long-term medication (longer than four weeks) may be given by district personnel provided that the prescribing physician completes the district medication permission request form.

Name of student ________________

Date of birth ________________ School ________________

To Be Completed by Physician

Name of medication ________________

Specific time(s) and dose(s) to be given at school ________________

Length of time ________________

Are there any restrictions? ___ yes ___ no If yes, what and how long? ____

____

________________ Printed Name of Physician

________________ Signature of Physician

________________ Date

To Be Completed by Parent

I, ________________, give permission for my child to receive the above medication as directed.

________________ Date

________________ Parent's/Guardian's Signature

________________ Telephone

MEDICAL SCREENING REFERRAL FORM

To the Parent or Guardian of ________________ D.O.B. ____________
(student's name)

As a result of the school Health Department's screening program, the following conditions have been found:

____
Date
____
Date
____
Date
____
Date

☐ The conditions listed above are not serious, and it is not necessary to see your doctor immediately. At your next regular visit, ask him or her about it. We suggest you have it checked no later than 3 6 9 months from now. (circle one)

☐ The conditions listed above should be examined by your doctor as soon as possible.

If you need more information or need help in locating a doctor, feel free to call your school nurse.

____
School Nurse Date

____
School Telephone Number

Doctor's Report to School Nurse (Please return as soon as possible)

Findings and recommendations given to parents ____________________

____

____

Are any modifications of the school program indicated? If so, what? ______

____

____

____

Do you wish to see the child again? If so, when? ____________________

______________________ ______________________
Physician's Printed Name Physician's Signature

______________________ ______________________
Office Telephone Number Date

DAILY REPORT FORM

DAILY REPORT FORM

NAME OF SCHOOL: ____________

DATE	IN TIME	STUDENT NAME	GRADE	TEACHER	Initial Visit	Follow-Up	Physical Assessment	Major Illness	Minor Illness	Emergency	First Aid	Emotional	Medication	Special Procedure	Child Abuse	Health Teaching	Health Counseling	Communicable Disease	Immunization	Other	Temperature	REASON	DISPOSITION: Back to Class	Parent Contact	Home	Physician	Hospital	Home Visit	Other	OUT TIME	SCREENING: Vision	Hearing	Weight & Height	Scalp/Skin	Blood Pressure	Dental	Scoliosis	Reportable Disease	T.B. Skin	Other	SIGNATURE & POSITION

WEIGHT - HEIGHT AVERAGES

	BOYS PERCENTILES 5th	50th	95th	AGE YRS.	GIRLS PERCENTILES 5th	50th	95th	
IN.	35	37¼	40¼	3.0	34½	37	39½	IN.
LB.	26½	32¼	39¼		25½	31	38	LB.
IN.	36½	39	41½	3.5	36	38½	41¼	IN.
LB.	28¼	34½	41½		27¼	33¼	41	LB.
IN.	37½	40¼	43¼	4.0	37½	40	42½	IN.
LB.	30	36½	44½		29	35¼	44	LB.
IN.	39	42	44½	4.5	38½	41¼	44	IN.
LB.	31½	39	47½		30½	37	46½	LB.
IN.	40¼	43¼	46	5.0	39½	42½	45½	IN.
LB.	33½	41¼	51		32	39	49½	LB.
IN.	41¼	44½	47¼	5.5	41	44	47	IN.
LB.	35½	43¼	54¼		33½	41	53¼	LB.
IN.	42½	45½	48½	6.0	42	45	48¼	IN.
LB.	37¼	45½	58		35½	43	56½	LB.
IN.	43½	46½	49½	6.5	43	46¼	49½	IN.
LB.	39¼	48	62		37¼	45¾	60½	LB.
IN.	44½	48	51	7.0	44	47½	51	IN.
LB.	41	50¼	66½		39	48¼	65½	LB.
IN.	45½	49	52¼	7.5	45	48½	52¼	IN.
LB.	43	53	71¼		41	51¼	70½	LB.
IN.	46½	50	53½	8.0	46	49½	53½	IN.
LB.	45	55½	76		43¼	54½	76½	LB.
IN.	47½	51	54½	8.5	47	51	55	IN.
LB.	47	58½	81½		45½	58½	82½	LB.
IN.	48½	52	55½	9.0	48	52	56¼	IN.
LB.	49	62	87¼		48	62½	89½	LB.
IN.	49¾	53	57	9.5	49¼	53¼	57½	IN.
LB.	51¼	65½	93¼		50½	67¼	96½	LB.
IN.	50¼	54½	58¼	10.0	50¼	54½	58½	IN.
LB.	53½	69¼	99½		53½	71½	104	LB.
IN.	51¼	55¼	59½	10.5	51¼	55½	60¼	IN.
LB.	56¼	73½	106½		56½	76½	111½	LB.
IN.	52¼	56½	61	11.0	52½	57	61½	IN.
LB.	59	77½	113½		60	81½	119	LB.
IN.	53¼	57½	62½	11.5	53½	58½	62½	IN.
LB.	62¼	82½	120½		63½	86½	126½	LB.
IN.	54¼	59	64	12.0	55	59½	64	IN.
LB.	65½	87½	128		67¼	91½	134	LB.
IN.	55¼	60¼	65½	12.5	56¼	60½	65¼	IN.
LB.	69½	93¼	135½		71¼	96½	141¼	LB.
IN.	56¼	61½	66½	13.0	57¼	61½	66¼	IN.
LB.	74¼	99	143¼		75¼	101½	148¼	LB.
IN.	57¼	63	68¼	13.5	58	62½	67	IN.
LB.	79	105½	151		79¼	106½	155	LB.
IN.	58½	64¼	69½	14.0	58½	63¼	67½	IN.
LB.	84¼	112	159		83¼	110½	161	LB.
IN.	59½	65½	70½	14.5	59	63½	67½	IN.
LB.	89½	118½	166½		87	114½	166½	LB.
IN.	61	66½	71½	15.0	59¼	63½	68	IN.
LB.	95	125	174½		90¼	118¼	171½	LB.
IN.	62¼	67½	72½	15.5	59½	63½	68¼	IN.
LB.	100¼	131¼	181½		93¼	121¼	175½	LB.
IN.	63½	68¼	73	16.0	59½	64	68¼	IN.
LB.	105¼	137	188½		95½	123¼	178½	LB.
IN.	64¼	69	73½	16.5	60	64	68¼	IN.
LB.	109½	142	195¼		97½	124½	180½	LB.
IN.	65	69¼	73½	17.0	60	64¼	68¼	IN.
LB.	113½	146¼	201¼		98½	125	181½	LB.
IN.	65¼	69½	73½	17.5	60¼	64¼	68¼	IN.
LB.	116½	149½	206½		99½	125	182¼	LB.
IN.	65¼	69½	73½	18.0	60½	64½	68¼	LB.
LB.	119	151½	211		99½	124½	181½	LB.

STUDENT TRANSFER RECORD

Student Transfer Record
Healthy Independent School District
Health Services Department
Immunization and Screening Data

Section CC-13.0
Record ALL Immunizations!

NAME (full) __________ Birth Date __________ Grade __________

Address __________ Telephone __________

Parent or Guardian __________

DPT or Td	Date #1	Date #2	Date #3	Date #4	Date #5	Date #6	Physician
Oral Polio	Date #1	Date #2	Date #3	Date #4	Date #5	Date #6	Physician

Rubeola	Date of Vaccine	Date of Disease	Physician
Rubella	Date of Vaccine		Physician
Mumps	Date of Vaccine	Date of Disease	Physician

Vision	R ______	L ______	Date of Test ______
Hearing	R ______	L ______	Date of Test ______

*Schools are reminded that transfer of immunization records (see Section BB-16.0) and screening results (see Section BB-32.0) ARE REQUIRED BY LAW.

HEPATITIS INFORMATION LETTER

Dear Parent:

A case of hepatitis has occurred in your child's classroom. We have taken the precautionary measures prescribed by the public health authorities to prevent the spread of the disease.

For your information, we would like to tell you what the American Academy of Pediatrics says about hepatitis: "It is a disease that is not very contagious (compared to measles, etc.) and therefore it is unusual for two cases to occur in the same classroom. It is usually mild in children. It is caused by a virus or germ that may be found in secretions of the mouth and nose, but is especially found in the urine and stool of the person with the disease. Therefore, washing the hands after going to the bathroom is especially important."

Protection with gamma globulin is recommended only for certain household contacts and people living in institutions such as orphanages or state hospitals.

If you have reason to believe that your child was exposed more intimately (spending the night at the home of the sick child, best friend, etc.) or if you have any other doubts or special questions, please call your family physician or contact the school nurse.

PERMANENT CUMULATIVE HEALTH RECORD, front Section CC-3.0

TAG FOR SPECIAL HEALTH CONDITION ______________________ *NOTE: All Referrals in Red Ink.*

Healthy Independent School District—Permanent Cumulative Health Record
Healthy, Texas

Parent Fill in Sections 1, 2, & 3 ONLY

1. Student's Name ______ (Last) ______ (First) ______ (M.I.) Date of Birth ____________ M___F___

2. Parent's Name ______________________ Address (in pencil) ______________________ Phone______

3. Student's Physical History:

	Year		Year
Accident—Serious		Neurological Disorder	
Allergy-Drug/Other		Orthopedic Handicap	
Asthma		Otitis Media	
Blood Disorder		Rheumatic Fever	
Cardiac Disease/Problem		Seizure Disorder	
Congenital Deformity		Speech Disorder	
Diabetes		Surgery—Serious	
Hearing Loss		T.B. Contact	
Hypertension		Ulcer	
Illness—Serious		Urinary Problem	
Kidney Disorder		Vision Loss	
Muscular Disorder		Other:	

GROWTH RECORD AND VISION

Date																				
Grade																				
Age																				
Height																				
Weight																				
Head Circumference																				
VISION	Type of Test																			
	Without Correction	R	20/	20/	20/	20/	20/	20/	20/	20/	20/	20/	20/	20/	20/	20/	20/	20/	20/	20/
		L	20/	20/	20/	20/	20/	20/	20/	20/	20/	20/	20/	20/	20/	20/	20/	20/	20/	20/
	Both Eyes		20/	20/	20/	20/	20/	20/	20/	20/	20/	20/	20/	20/	20/	20/	20/	20/	20/	20/
	With Correction (Glasses or Contacts)	R	20/	20/	20/	20/	20/	20/	20/	20/	20/	20/	20/	20/	20/	20/	20/	20/	20/	20/
		L	20/	20/	20/	20/	20/	20/	20/	20/	20/	20/	20/	20/	20/	20/	20/	20/	20/	20/

IMMUNIZATION RECORD

Prevention Record	1st Dose Mo/Yr	2nd Dose Mo/Yr	3rd Dose Mo/Yr	Booster Mo/Yr	Booster Mo/Yr
Diphtheria/Pertussis/ Tetanus					
Tetanus/Diphtheria					
Polio					
Rubeola (Vac. or Date/Illness					
Rubella					
Mumps (Vac. or Date/Illness					
MMR					
TB Test					
Chest X-Ray					
Other					
Verifying Physician/Clinic					
Nurse/Signature					

Medical/Religious Exemption:

Physician Recommendations, Restrictions, Medications

Reason	Dates

HYPERTENSION SCREENING

Date													
R													
L													

Special Services: Recommendations, Reports, Program Adjustment

***DENTAL SCREENING**

Date	Results	Referred	Corrected	Re-Ck

*Code

*C-Caries; G-Gingivitis; H-Hygiene; O-Orthodontic; O.K.-No problem

PERMANENT CUMULATIVE HEALTH RECORD, back

NAME | D.O.B. | *NOTE: All Referrals in Red Ink.*

TEACHER OBSERVATION

Use X when defect observed; circle X when corrected

H.I.—Record health inventory in first TNC column

Teacher-Nurse Conference Date		HI									
General	Tires easily										
	Under or overweight										
	Posture										
	Muscular coordination										
	Hair, Scalp, Skin										
	Personal hygiene										
Eyes	Eyelids										
	Strabismus										
	Squint										
	Frequent headaches										
	Eyes water										
Ears	Discharge										
	Earaches										
	Does not hear well										
Nose	Freq. colds—nosebleeds										
Mouth	Mouth breathing										
Throat	Freq. sore throat										
Teeth	Oral hygiene										
	Obvious defects										
	Gums										
Behavior Pattern	Disturbs classroom										
	Nervous/restless										
	Twitching—fainting										
	Nail biting										
	Shy										
	Over-agressiveness										
	Freq. stomachaches										
	Excessive use of toilet										
	Peer relations										
	Doesn't like school										
Other	Food habits										
	Speech Problem										
	General Cleanliness										
	Excessive Absence										

Date	Referral and Follow-Up	Nurse

Audiometric Screening

Date	Sweep Norm	Freq.	250	500	1000	2000	3000	4000	6000
	R	R db							
	L	L db							
	R	R db							
	L	L db							
	R	R db							
	L	L db							
	R	R db							
	L	L db							
	R	R db							
	L	L db							
	R	R db							
	L	L db							
	R	R db							
	L	L db							
	R	R db							
	L	L db							

(AUDIOGRAM spans 250–6000.)

Scoliosis Screening

Date	Key	Finding - Correction	Nurse

P-Passed, Re-Ck, F-Failed, R-Referred

REPORT OF VISION/HEARING SCREENING EXAMINATION, front

To the parents of ______________________________ Date of Birth ______________
STUDENT/S NAME

A recent VISION/HEARING screening examination showed that your child should be checked more thoroughly
(CIRCLE ONE)

by a VISION/HEARING Specialist.
(CIRCLE ONE)

If you have any questions or need any help, feel free to consult with the school nurse.

See reverse side for results of screening.

______________________ ______________________
SCHOOL NURSE SCHOOL

______________________ ______________________
DATE TELEPHONE NO.

SPECIALIST'S REPORT TO SCHOOL NURSE

In addition to your medical diagnosis, will you please detail for the classroom teacher any modifications of the regular school program that may be helpful in this student's education. (E.g. special seating, repetition of instruction, special materials, etc.)

____

____

____

____

____

______________________ ______________________
PHYSICIAN'S PRINTED NAME PHYSICIAN'S SIGNATURE

______________________ ______________________
OFFICE PHONE DATE

Rev. 3/83

REPORT OF VISION/HEARING SCREENING EXAMINATION, back

____
STUDENT'S NAME

Note to: VISION/HEARING Specialist
(CIRCLE ONE)

The above child has been referred because of:

☐ A primary defect discovered during routine screening exams

☐ A learning problem which may be related to a visual or auditory problem

☐ Other ______________________

____

Results of Vision Screening Exam:

Visual Acuity: Test Method Used

Without Glasses R. ______ L. ______ Snellen 10′ ______ 20′ ______

With Glasses R. ______ L. ______ Titmus ______

Other ______

Latent Hyperopia (+2.5 lens)

☐ passed ☐ failed ☐ not tested

Muscle Imbalance (cover test)

☐ passed ☐ failed ☐ not tested

Other ______________________

____

Results of Hearing Screening Exam:

Impedance Bridge Screening:

☐ Abnormal ☐ normal ☐ not performed

Audiogram (attached)

R ☐ passed ☐ failed ☐ not performed

L ☐ passed ☐ failed ☐ nor performed

Other ______________________

____

DAILY LOG FOR MEDICATION

Daily Log for Medication

School	Week of					Week of					Week of					Week of				
	Mon	Tue	Wed	Thu	Fri	Mon	Tue	Wed	Thu	Fri	Mon	Tue	Wed	Thu	Fri	Mon	Tue	Wed	Thu	Fri
Student ______ Med. ______ Dosage ______ Times ______																				
Student ______ Med. ______ Dosage ______ Times ______																				
Student ______ Med. ______ Dosage ______ Times ______																				
Student ______ Med. ______ Dosage ______ Times ______																				
Student ______ Med. ______ Dosage ______ Times ______																				
Student ______ Med. ______ Dosage ______ Times ______																				
Student ______ Med. ______ Dosage ______ Times ______																				

The person dispensing the medication signs his or her name in the block under the corresponding day of the week.

PHYSICIAN'S AUTHORIZATION FOR HAVING SPECIALIZED PHYSICAL HEALTH CARE SERVICE PROCEDURES ADMINISTERED

Name of Student: ______________________ Birth Date ______________

Address: ____

1. Physical condition for which the standardized procedure is to be performed: ______________

____

2. Name of standardized procedure: ______________________________

3. Precautions, possible untoward reactions, and interventions: ______________

____

____

4. Time schedule and/or indication for the procedure: ______________________

____

5. The procedure is to be continued as above until: ______________________
(Date)

______________________________ ______________
Physician's Signature Date

______________________________ ______________
Address Telephone

I hereby request that the treatment specified above be performed to the above-named child.

______________________________ ______________
Signature of Parent/Guardian Date

STUDENT EMERGENCY CARD, front

Student Emergency Card

Date ____________
School ____________
Grade ____________
Birth Date ____________

Student's Name ______________________________
Last First Middle

Address ______________________________ Home Telephone ____________
City ______________________ Zip ____________

TO PARENT OR GUARDIAN: To serve your child in case of ACCIDENT OR SUDDEN ILLNESS, it is necessary that you furnish the following information for emergency calls:

Name **Business Address** **Business Telephone**

Mother ______________________________
Father ______________________________

LIST TWO NEIGHBORS OR NEARBY RELATIVES WHO WILL ASSUME TEMPORARY CARE OF YOUR CHILD IF YOU CANNOT BE REACHED:

Name ____________________ Name ____________________
Address ______________ Tel ________ Address ______________ Tel ________

HEALTH INFORMATION: List any health conditions such as heart disease, diabetes, epilepsy, severe allergies, eye or ear problems, or any chronic condition, etc.

Explanation: ______________________________
____

DOCTOR: 1st choice ____________________ 2nd choice ____________________
Telephone Number ____________________ Telephone Number ____________________
HOSPITAL CHOICE: Address ______________________________ Telephone Number ____________

IMPORTANT—PLEASE COMPLETE REVERSE SIDE OF CARD

STUDENT EMERGENCY CARD, back

(Back of Emergency Card)

I, the undersigned, do hereby authorize officials of ______________________ School District to contact directly the persons named on this card, and do authorize the named physicians to render such treatment as may be deemed necessary in an emergency, for the health of said child.

In the event physicians, other persons named on this card, or parents cannot be contacted, the school officials are hereby authorized to take whatever action is deemed necessary in their judgment, for the health of the aforesaid child.

I will not hold the school district financially responsible for the emergency care and/or transportation for said child.

____
Signature of Parent or Guardian

____
Student's Last Name First Initial

ACCIDENT REPORT

To be filled in at the time of the accident by the person caring for an injured student who is referred to a docter:

Student name ______________________ Phone ______________

Address ______________________ Age ______ Sex ______

Date ______________ Time ______________ Insurance ______________

Grade ______ Teacher ______________ School ______________

Location of accident ______________________

Person in attendance ______________________

Nature of Accident	
Abrasion	Head Injury
Bruise/Bump	Fracture
Burn	Laceration
Cut	Puncture
Convulsion	Shock
Dislocation	Sprain

Other ______________________

Part of Body Injured		
Abdomen	Eye*	Head
Ankle*	Face	Knee*
Arm*	Finger*	Leg*
Back	Foot*	Teeth
Chest	Hand	Wrist*
Elbow*		

Other ______________________

*Left, right, both

How did it happen? ______________________

____

____

____

Were parents notified? Yes ______ No ______

Treatment and disposition: ______________________

____

Follow-up: ______________________

Amount of time lost from school: ______________________

(Signature) ______________________
Principal, Teacher, or Nurse

HEAD INJURY SHEET

Dear Parent:

Today, ____________(Child's Name)____________ received an injury to the head. Your child was seen in the clinic and had no problems at that time, but you should watch for any of the following symptoms:

1. Severe headache.
2. Excessive drowsiness (awake the child at least twice during the night).
3. Nausea and/or vomiting.
4. Double vision, blurred vision, or pupils of different sizes.
5. Loss of muscle coordination such as falling down, walking strangely, or staggering.
6. Any unusual behavior such as being confused, breathing irregularly, or being dizzy.
7. Convulsion.
8. Bleeding or discharge from an ear.

CONTACT YOUR LOCAL DOCTOR OR EMERGENCY ROOM IF YOU NOTICE ANY OF THE ABOVE SYMPTOMS.

____
School Nurse

____
Telephone Number

ANIMAL BITE RECORD

Date of bite: ______________________ Time of bite: ______________________

Name of person involved: ______________________

Address: ______________________

City, State, Zip: ______________________

Telephone: ______________________ Age: __________ Sex: __________

Breed/Type of animal with general description: ______________________

____

Age of animal: ______________________ Sex of animal: ______________________

Approximate weight of animal: ______________________

Date of vaccination: ______________________ City: ______________________

Description of incident (on school grounds? to/from school? animal confined, leashed/unleashed? etc.) __________

____

Area on person bitten: ______________________

Owner of animal: ______________________

Address: ______________________

City, State, Zip: ______________________

Telephone: ______________________

Bite reported to: (LOCAL ANIMAL CONTROL AGENCY)

Time & Date reported: ______________________

Signature: ______________________

SCHOOL HEALTH PROGRAM
LETTER TO PARENT

School ______________________________ Date ____________

Name of Child ______________________________ Grade ________

Name of Teacher ______________________________

Dear Parent:

In watching the health of your child, the teacher and I have noted the following observations which we feel should be brought to your attention:

____

____

____

____

______________	______________	______________
Principal	Nurse	Phone

The school would appreciate comments from you or your doctor regarding these signs if you feel the information would be helpful for the nurse or teacher.

Date: ______________________

Parent's comments <u>OR</u> Doctor's diagnosis, treatment, and recommendations:

____

____

____

____

____

______________		______________
Parent's Signature	OR	Doctor's Signature

BIBLIOGRAPHICAL REFERENCES

Accardo, P. J., and A. J. Capute. *The Pediatrician and the Developmentally Delayed Child.* Baltimore: University Park Press, 1979.

Ayers, A. J. "Improving Academic Scores through Sensory Integration." *Journal of Learning Disabilities* 5:339, 1972.

Barlos, D. "Sexually Transmitted Disease." *The Facts.* New York: Oxford University Press, 1979.

Bergsma, D. *Birth Defects Compendium;* 2nd edition. White Plains, N.Y.: Alan R. Liss, Inc., 1979.

Cott, A. "Megavitamins. The Orthomolecular Approach to Behavioral Disorders and Learning Disability." *Academic Therapy* 7:245–58, 1972.

Cruikshank, W. M. *Learning Disabilities in Home, School, and Community.* Syracuse: Syracuse University Press, 1977.

De Angelis, Catherine. *Pediatric Primary Care.* Boston: Little, Brown and Company, 1979.

Diagnostic and Statistical Manual of Mental Disorders III. Washington: American Psychiatric Association, 1980.

Doman, R. J., et al. "Children with Severe Brain Injury; Neurologic Organization in Terms of Mobility." *JAMA* 174:257–62, 1966.

Faas, Larry A. *The Emotionally Disturbed Child.* Springfield: C. C. Thomas, 1975.

Feigin, R. D., and J. D. Cherry. *Textbook of Pediatric Infectious Diseases.* Philadelphia: W. B. Saunders Company, 1981.

Feingold, B. *Why Your Child Is Hyperactive.* New York: Random House, 1975.

Golden, G. S. "Nonstandard Therapies in Developmental Disabilities." *American Journal of Disease of Children* 134:487–91, 1980.

Gubbay, S. S. *The Clumsy Child.* Philadelphia: W. B. Saunders Company, 1975.

Helfer. R. E. *Childhood Comes First.* Lansing: R. E. Helfer, 1978.

Hervett, Frank M. "Strategies of Special Education." *Pediatric Clinics of North America* 20, no. 3, 1973.

Kempe, C. H., and R. E. Helfer. *Helping the Battered Child and His Family.* Philadelphia: Lippincott, 1972.

Kephart, N. C. *The Slow Learner in the Classroom.* Columbus: Charles Merrill, 1960.

King, A., and C. Nicol. *Venereal Disease,* 3rd edition. Baltimore: Williams and Wilkins, 1975.

Kinsbourne, M., and P. J. Caplan. *Children's Learning and Attention Problems.* Boston: Little, Brown and Company, 1979.

Kovacs, M., and A. T. Beck. "An Empirical Clinical Approach toward a Definition of Childhood Depression." In J. G. Schulterbrandt and A. Raskin (eds.), *Depression in Children, Diagnosis, Treatment, and Conceptual Models.* New York: Rowan Press, 1977.

Lazar, P. "Hair Analysis: What Does It Tell Us?" *JAMA* 229:1908–9, 1974.

Lefkowits, M. M., and N. Burton. *Psychological Bulletin* 85, no. 4, 716–26.

Lerner, J. *Children with Learning Disabilities,* 2nd edition. Boston: Houghton Mifflin, 1976.

Levine, M. D., and J. P. Shankoff. *A Pediatric Approach to Learning Disabilities.* New York: John Wiley and Sons, 1980.

Morbidity and Mortality Weekly Report, Rabies Prevention, U.S. Dept. of Health and Human Services, June 13, 1980.

Murdek, G. C. "The Abused Child and the School System," *American Journal of Public Health,* 60:105–9, 1970.

Paluzny, Maria J. *Autism: A Practical Guide for Parents and Professionals.* Syracuse: Syracuse University Press, 1979.

Parcel, Guy. *Teaching My Parents about Asthma.* Galveston: University of Texas Medical Branch, 1976.

Paulson, M. M., D. Stone, and R. Sposto. "Suicide Potential in Children Ages 4 to 12." *Suicide and Life-Threatening Behavior,* 8:225–42.

Philpott, W. H., et al. "Allergic States in Children with Learning Problems." Read before the Ninth International Congress of ACLD. Atlantic City, N.J., February 1972.

Rutter, M. "Diagnosis and Definition of Childhood Autism." *Journal of Autism and Childhood Schizophrenia* 8:139–61, June 1978.

Safer, D. J., and R. P. Allen. *Hyperactive Children.* Baltimore: University Park Press, 1976.

Silver, L. B "Acceptable and Controversial Approaches to Treating Learning Disability." *Pediatrics* 55:406–15, 1975.

Symposium on Child Abuse, Supplement to *Pediatrics,* April 1973, vol. 51, no. 4.

Vaughan, D., and T. Asbury. *General Ophthalmology,* 8th edition. Los Altos, CA: Lange Medical Publications, 1977.

Vaughn, V. C., R. J. McKay, and R. E. Behrman. *Nelson Textbook of Pediatrics,* 11th edition. Philadelphia: W. B. Saunders Company, 1979.

Weston, H. C. *Sight, Light, and Efficiency.* London: H. K. Lewis and Company, 1949.

Wiederhold, J. "Historical Perspectives on the Education of the Learning Disabled." In L. Mann and D. Sabatino (eds.), *The Second Review of Special Education.* Philadelphia: Journal of Special Education Press, 1974.

INDEX